ECG Manual for the
VETERINARY TECHNICIAN

ECG Manual for the VETERINARY TECHNICIAN

N. JOEL EDWARDS, D.V.M.
Diplomate American College of
Veterinary Internal Medicine
(Cardiology)
Albany, New York

Adjunct Associate Professor of Medicine
Department of Clinical Sciences
New York State College of Veterinary
Medicine
Cornell University, Ithaca, New York

W.B. SAUNDERS COMPANY ———————— **Harcourt Brace Jovanovich, Inc.**
Philadelphia   London   Toronto   Montreal   Sydney   Tokyo

W. B. SAUNDERS COMPANY
Harcourt Brace Jovanovich, Inc.

The Curtis Center
Independence Square West
Philadelphia, PA 19106

Library of Congress Cataloging-in-Publication Data
Edwards, N. Joel
    ECG manual for the veterinary technician / N. Joel Edwards. — 1st
ed.
        p.   cm.
    ISBN 0-7216-3083-9
    1. Veterinary electrocardiography — Handbooks, manuals, etc.
I. Title.
SF811.E39   1993
636.089'61207547 — dc20   92-25705

ECG MANUAL for the VETERINARY TECHNICIAN   ISBN 0-7216-3083-9

Printed in the United States of America.

Last digit is the print number: 9   8   7   6   5   4   3   2   1

Preface

The use of clinical electrocardiography in veterinary medicine is becoming an increasingly routine portion of the patient data base. It has been estimated by some that as many as 10% of all patients being attended to by a veterinarian can be helped by information gained from an electrocardiogram (ECG).

The first recorded use of electrocardiography in animals occurred in 1887 when Augustus D. Waller used his pet bulldog, Jimmie, in his early ECG studies in humans. Since that time, normal values have been established for many animals, including the dog, cat, cow, horse, pig, ferret, sheep, and goat. This text focuses predominantly on the dog and cat, with some examples for the horse, cow, and ferret. Additional pages focus on understanding basic physiology of the cardiac conduction system; producing a readable, artifact-free electrocardiogram; identifying and measuring all wave forms; and recognizing the more significant dysrhythmias. Where applicable, appropriate response measures are discussed.

In today's veterinary practice, the veterinary technician is contributing more and more toward the effective "team" management of veterinary patients. This, of course, includes the cardiac patient. Each and every veterinary technician should have a basic understanding of cardiac physiology, be able to record an artifact-free ECG, understand how to make the ECG measurements, and, in most instances, be able to recognize life-threatening arrhythmias.

Learning how to use the information gained from an ECG or surgical monitor depicting the ECG tracing is not difficult if one is willing to follow a systematic method of evaluation. Once the principles are understood, they may be applied to any species under any condition.

The purpose of this text is to provide instruction for veterinary technicians in electrocardiography. Examples of normal ECG recordings, practice ECGs, and examples of various ECG abnormalities will help the reader to feel comfortable and confident around the ECG. Review questions and self-assessment sections allow readers to utilize their own thought processes in clinical simulations.

With little effort, each reader should find between these covers some enlightenment, some practical understanding of electrocardiography, and, most important of all, some fun.

The workbook format is designed to facilitate easy learning and return visits to the pages. Writing this manual has been a reflection of my respect and admiration for veterinary technicians as a group and, in particular, those dedicated men and women with whom I have had the privilege of working side by side over the years.

N. JOEL EDWARDS, D.V.M.

Acknowledgments

Without the help and guidance of our fellow beings, one alone becomes no one. So too it is only with the help of others that this work was born.

First and foremost, I am indebted to my wife, Cinnia, for rescuing the manuscript in the midst of her own pursuit of a nursing career, computer changes, and an acute appendectomy. Without illustrations, the written word lacks enlightenment. Thanks go to Amy S. Edwards and Jane S. Jorgensen for their wonderful illustrations and to Amy S. Edwards for her redrawing of several of the ECG tracings. I would also like to thank Elizabeth Peck, LVT, and Lori Grant, LVT, for their review and constructive criticism of the manuscript. My appreciation also goes to my fellow veterinarians who have contributed material and offered support, encouragement, and intellectual stimulation, particularly Donald Dries and Lawrence W. Bartholf.

I am indebted to the production and editing departments of W. B. Saunders Company, particularly to Darlene Pedersen, Senior Vice President and Editorial Director, who had the courage to undertake the concept, and to Selma Ozmat, Editor of Veterinary Technology, whose patience and encouragement were extremely supportive, and to Scott Weaver and Bill Preston for their technical support.

N. JOEL EDWARDS, D.V.M.

Contents

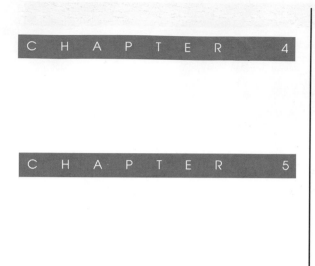

Key Words and Concepts

1

Basic Principles of Electrocardiography

GENERAL OVERVIEW

The science of electrocardiography encompasses the recording of electrical activity generated by the heart. This electrical activity is recorded on the surface of the body via electrodes that are attached at various positions on the body (Fig. 1–1). These electrodes transmit the electrical information to a machine called an electrocardiograph, which produces a recording either on a monitor screen or on paper, which is called an electrocardiogram (ECG). This enables the viewer to see a pictorial representation of both the amplitude (amount of electrical activity) and the duration (length of time) of this electrical activity. Each mechanical contraction of the heart (heart rate) is preceded by an electrical wavefront (potential differences of electrical current) that stimulates heart muscle contraction followed by relaxation in preparation for the next heart beat. The stimulus for contraction, precipitated primarily by a movement of sodium ions into the cell, is termed "depolarization." Relaxation, precipitated principally by the movement of sodium and potassium ions back out of the cell, is called "repolarization." The currents generated by this movement of ions in and out of cardiac cells are what constitute the visible ECG tracing as they are recorded on paper or seen on a monitor.

As you might imagine, this electrical activity is highly organized and rhythmic occurring in an orderly, repeatable fashion. As the electrical current (wavefront) travels from its point of origin, the sinoatrial node, to its final destination in the muscle cells of the ventricles (ventricular myocardial cells) continuous wave forms are recorded on the ECG. This continuous waveform has different parts, which have been labeled by early scientists as P, Q, R, S, and T waves (Fig. 1–2). Each wave represents the electrical activity that occurs in different parts of the heart during depolarization and repolarization of heart cells.

Under normal circumstances, the electrical sequence that triggers each heartbeat begins in a small strip of specialized cardiac tissue, called the sinoatrial node (S-A node) located in the right atrium. The firing of the S-A node sends electrical impulses through the atria (upper chambers of the heart), causing atrial depolarization, creating the P waves on the ECG and triggering atrial contraction. The impulses then travel through the atrioventricular node (A-V node), bundle of His, right and left bundle branches, Purkinje fibers, and ventricular muscle cells, causing ventricular depolarization and creating the Q, R, and S waves (QRS complex) on the ECG and triggering ventricular contraction (Fig. 1–3). The T wave is formed when the ventricles return to their resting state (ventricular repolarization).

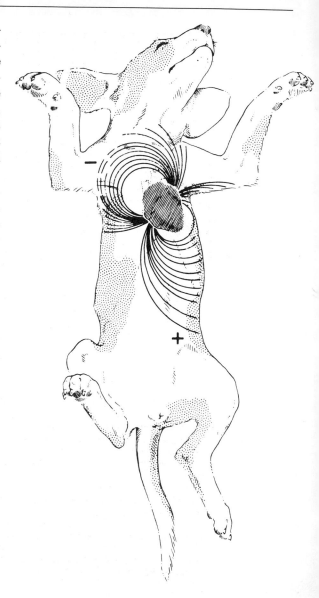

Figure 1–1 ■ The tissues and body fluids surrounding the heart conduct electrical currents easily. These impulses can be sensed, amplified, and recorded on the ECG via electrodes attached to skin on the legs. (From Edwards, NJ: Bolton's Handbook of Canine and Feline Electrocardiography, ed 2. Philadelphia, WB Saunders, 1987, with permission.)

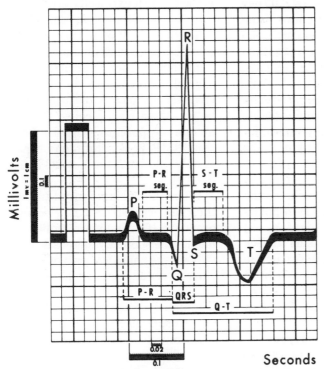

Figure 1-2 ■ This shows a normal lead II electrocardiographic complex. The electrocardiograph has been standardized at 1 cm = 1 mv, so that each small box on the vertical axis equals 0.1 mv. This tracing was recorded at 50 mm/sec paper speed, so each small box on the horizontal axis equals 0.02 sec.

Atrial depolarization is indicated by the P wave. Following the P wave there is a short delay in the A-V node (P-R segment), after which the ventricles depolarize and produce the QRS complex. Ths S-T segment and the T wave represent ventricular repolarization. (From Edwards, NJ: Bolton's Handbook of Canine and Feline Electrocardiography, ed 2. Philadelphia, WB Saunders, 1987, with permission.)

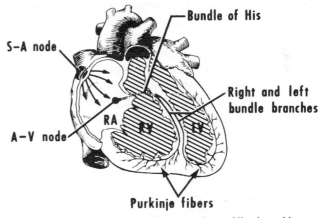

Figure 1-3 ■ The conduction system of the heart includes the S-A node, the interatrial bundles, the A-V node, the bundle of His and its branches, and the Purkinje fibers. The S-A node lies in the right atrium, and atrial conduction occurs at the rate of 500 to 1000 mm/sec. Conduction through the A-V node is slow (100 mm/sec), which allows the atria to empty into the ventricles before ventricular contraction occurs. The Purkinje fibers conduct rapidly (2000 mm/sec) and terminate in the myocardium. Muscle cell-to-muscle cell transmission occurs where the Purkinje fibers terminate, and the conduction across the ventricular muscle cells occurs at the rate of 400 mm/sec. (From Edwards, NJ: Bolton's Handbook of Canine and Feline Electrocardiography, ed 2. Philadelphia, WB Saunders, 1987, with permission.)

It is the assessment of the shape, height (amplitude), and width (duration) of these wave forms (P, Q, R, S, T) and the intervals between the waveforms (P-R and S-T) (review Fig. 1–2) that is the science of electrocardiography. It is here that the veterinary technician can, by understanding the normal and distinguishing the abnormal, directly contribute to the care and treatment of the cardiac patient. This will become particularly important in the recognition of life-threatening dysrhythmias (irregular heartbeats). It is also important to understand that the ECG is a measure of electrical activity only, having no reference to the mechanical performance (pumping ability) of the heart. Before proceeding further, it is important to review the cellular physiology that accounts for this phenomenon.

CELLULAR PHYSIOLOGY AND THE GENERATION OF ELECTRICAL IMPULSES

Electrical activity in the heart is produced by a series of pacemaker cells (S-A nodal cells) with rapid discharge and cells with progressively slower discharge rates throughout the rest of the system, leading eventually to electrical stimulation of myocardial cells, which triggers mechanical contraction. The system is also equipped with a kind of fail-safe mechanism, whereby cells farther down in the system (below the S-A node) such as the A-V node or

Purkinje fibers will fire off on their own if they do not receive an electrical stimulus from higher up in the system. Take a moment and review Figure 1–3. Each of these areas will be covered in more detail later in this chapter. First, however, the transmembrane ionic movement of sodium ions (Na^+), potassium ions (K^+), calcium ions (Ca^{2+}), and chloride ions (Cl^-) into and out of cells responsible for the generation of electrical current must be understood.

Cardiac muscle cell physiology is similar in many ways to that of other muscle cells. In the normal resting state the cell is said to be polarized. In this polarized state the inside of the cell is negative with respect to the outside surface (Fig. 1–4A). The polarity is maintained by the distribution and concentration of intracellular and extracellular ions. The cell membrane is primarily responsible for the manner in which these ions are distributed.

The resting cell membrane is nearly impermeable to sodium ions (Na^+) and is partially permeable to potassium (K^+) and chloride (Cl^-) ions. In addition, there is a metabolic cellular "pump" within the cell membrane that actively pumps Na^+ out of the cell. The concentration of Na^+ is much higher extracellularly because of the sodium pump and because the cell membrane will not allow sodium to diffuse into the cell. The concentration of K^+ is much higher intracellularly than extracellularly (about 20:1), which favors the diffusion of K^+ out of the cell through the partially permeable cell membrane. The concentration of Cl^-

is the greatest extracellularly, which favors the diffusion of Cl^- into the cell.

The net result of all these forces is a greater number of negative charges inside the cell and a greater number of positive charges outside the cell. The relative difference between the charges on each side of the cell membrane can be measured and is called the resting transmembrane potential (RMP) (see Fig. 1–5). The RMP is constant and equals approximately −90 mv in the normal healthy myocardial cell.

When the cell is polarized and the ions are in their respective places, no electrical current is produced. If a stimulus is applied to the cell, the membrane suddenly increases its permeability to Na^+, and there is a rush of Na^+ into the cell. This causes a temporary reversal of intracellular charges (Fig. 1–4B). After the cell has been stimulated to depolarize, the depolarization process spreads rapidly along the entire length of the muscle fiber without additional stimulation. This wave of shifting ions produces a measurable electrical current (Fig. 1–4B). Inward movements of Cl^- during phase 1 and of Ca^{2+} during phase 2 of the myocardial action potential also contribute to the ionic shifts responsible for depolarization. The magnitude of the electrical forces produced is proportional to the length and diameter of the muscle fiber and to the relative resistivity of the conducted medium (blood) — the Brody effect. It is for this reason that dilatation (lengthening of the muscle fibers) and hypertrophy (thickening of the muscle fibers) cause an increase in elec-

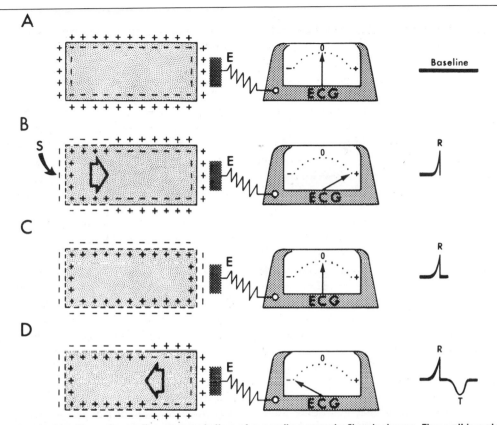

Figure 1-4 ■ *A*, A resting schematic representation of a cardiac muscle fiber is shown. The cell is polarized, which means that the outside of the cell is positive with respect to the inside, owing to the distribution of extracellular and intracellular ions. In this polarized state, there is no electrical activity, and the electrode (E), which is attached to the body surface, records a steady straight baseline. *B*, Upon stimulation (*S* with *curved arrow*), the fiber begins to depolarize. There is a sudden shift of ions, and the charges reverse themselves. This depolarization process spreads along the entire length of the fiber (*open arrow*), the electrode (E) detects a wave of electrical current flowing toward it, and it records a positive deflection (R) on the electrocardiogram. *C*, Once the entire fiber has been depolarized, the electrical current no longer flows, and the tracing returns to the baseline. *D*, Repolarization begins as the ions gradually return to their original positions. As repolarization of the entire fiber proceeds, another wave of electrical current flows. In this instance the current is flowing away from the electrode (E), and a negative deflection occurs (T). The T wave can be positive or negative in most leads. (From Edwards, NJ: Bolton's Handbook of Canine and Feline Electrocardiography, ed 2. Philadelphia, WB Saunders, 1987, with permission.)

trical forces that can be measured on the ECG.

Shortly after the cell membrane becomes permeable to Na^+ and depolarizes, it becomes much more permeable to K^+, and K^+ begins to leave the cell. At this point, repolarization begins (Fig. 1-4*C*). Repolarization occurs much more slowly than depolarization. The cell membrane regains its impermeable state, and most of the repolarization depends on the gradual removal of Na^+ from the cell by the sodium-potassium pump mechanism. The shifting of ions during repolarization also produces a measurable electrical current (Fig. 1-4*D*). When this abrupt shifting of ions during depolarization and repolarization takes place across the cardiac muscle cell membrane, an action potential is generated that stimulates mechanical contraction. Although it is thought that calcium movement into the myofibrils catalyzes the excitation-contraction-coupling event, the precise mechanism by which the electrical impulses initiate muscular contraction is still unknown.

The membrane action potential can be recorded by placing an electrode inside a cell and then recording the changes in electrical potential that occur across the membrane at the exact point (Fig. 1-5). The depolarization wave starts at that point and continues for the length of the muscle fiber. The threshold potential (TP) determines the ease with which a muscle fiber can be stimulated. A stimulatory impulse must be strong enough to exceed the TP before depolarization will begin. Diseases

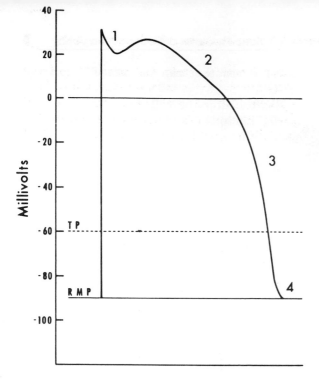

Figure 1–5 ■ A myocardial membrane action potential is measured by placing an electrode inside a muscle cell and then recording the changes in electrical potential that occur across the membrane at that point. The resting membrane potential (RMP) indicates that the inside of the resting cell is about −90 mv, more negative than the outside. If the cell is stimulated an action potential occurs, causing depolarization, so that the cell suddenly is more positive intracellularly. During phases 2 and 3 the intracellular electronegativity is gradually restored and, during phase 4, the fiber is again resting. Whenever the threshold potential (TP) is exceeded, an action potential occurs and causes depolarization of the entire muscle fiber. (From Edwards, NJ: Bolton's Handbook of Canine and Feline Electrocardiography, ed 2. Philadelphia, WB Saunders, 1987, with permission.)

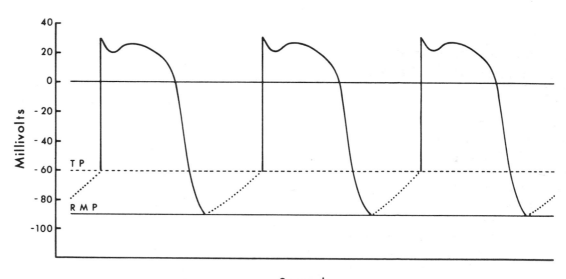

Figure 1–6 ■ Shown here is the typical action potential of a specialized cardiac pacemaker fiber (Purkinje tissue). Unlike the other fibers, which remain at the RMP, the pacemaker tissues can depolarize automatically. During phase 4 of their action potential, Na+ gradually leaks into the fiber, and the intracellular space becomes less and less negative until the TP is reached, an action potential occurs, and the fiber discharges an impulse that is propagated along the conduction pathway to other muscle fibers. The RMP and the TP of pacemaker cells differ at various points in the heart. (From Edwards, NJ: Bolton's Handbook of Canine and Feline Electrocardiography, ed 2. Philadelphia, WB Saunders, 1987, with permission.)

or drugs that alter cell membrane permeability, conduction velocity, RMP, or TP will alter the sensitivity of the cell. For example, the antiarrhythmic drug quinidine works in part by increasing the TP, making the cells less sensitive to stimulation and less prone to produce dysrhythmias.

SPECIAL PHYSIOLOGIC PROPERTIES OF CARDIAC MUSCLE CELLS

The electrical activity in the heart is highly organized. The electrical excitation of the heart is rhythmic, and occurs rapidly in an orderly sequence. Several characteristics that cardiac muscle cells possess allow for such fine coordination including automaticity, conductivity, and excitability.

Certain specialized cardiac tissues can depolarize automatically, without an outside stimulus. These tissues, called the pacemaker tissues, are said to possess automaticity, or the ability to discharge spontaneously. They have automaticity because of a difference in their cell membranes' permeability to Na^+ and K^+. During phase 4 of the action potential, represented by the dotted lines between the RMP and the TP shown in Figure 1–6, Na^+ leaks into the cell and raises the electrical potential to the TP. This initiates an action potential, and depolarization begins. Pacemaker tissues are located in the S-A node, junctional fibers (specialized atrial fibers in the area of the A-V node), bundle of His and its branches, and

Purkinje fibers. Under extreme conditions, other atrial and ventricular muscle fibers are capable of automaticity.

The rate at which each of these pacemaker tissues automatically discharges is different.

The S-A node normally has the most rapid rate of spontaneous depolarization (generally 70 to 160 times/minute for the dog and 160 to 240 times/minute for the cat), and consequently it is the usual cardiac pacemaker (Fig. 1–7). If

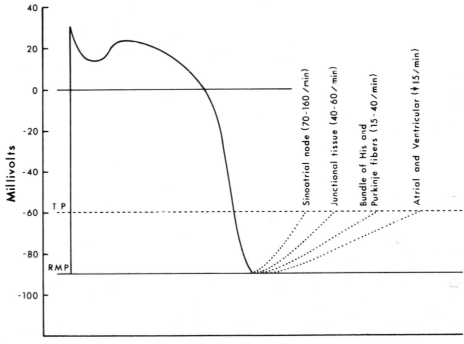

Figure 1–7 ▪ Different rates of automatic discharge of the various cardiac pacemaker tissues are shown. The S-A node is the usual cardiac pacemaker, because it has the most rapid rate of spontaneous depolarization (70 to 160 times per minute). If the S-A node were to become inactive, the junctional tissues in the area of the A-V node would pace the heart at 40 to 60 beats per minute. If both the S-A node and the junctional fibers were to become inactive, the bundle of His or the Purkinje fibers could pace the heart at 15 to 40 times per minute. Under extreme conditions the atrial and ventricular fibers may discharge at very slow rates, serving as a last-ditch measure to maintain life. (*Solid dark line* represents the action potential of a myocardial cell; *dotted lines* show relative rates of spontaneous discharge. See Figure 1–8 for a more accurate representation of the various action potentials.) (From Edwards, NJ: Bolton's Handbook of Canine and Feline Electrocardiography, ed 2. Philadelphia, WB Saunders, 1987, with permission.)

the S-A node were to become inactivated, the junctional tissues would have the next most rapid rate of automatic discharge (40 to 60 times/minute), and they would subsequently act as the cardiac pacemaker (Fig. 1–7). If both the S-A tissues and the junctional tissues become inactivated, the bundle of His, its branches, or the Purkinje fibers would pace the heart at 15 to 40 beats/minute (Fig. 1–7). If all the other pacemaker tissues fail, atrial or ventricular muscle fibers can discharge on their own at very slow rates (Fig. 1–7). These rates are somewhat higher in the cat, although the relationship is the same as in the dog. The various cardiac tissues have differently shaped action potentials (Fig. 1–8). Their relationship to the surface ECG is depicted in Figures 1–9 and 1–10.

Another important concept of cardiac muscle cell physiology is the functional syncytium principle, or the "all-or-none" phenomenon. There are two main functional syncytia—the atrial syncytium and the ventricular syncytium. They communicate through the A-V node and bundle of His. Otherwise, the atrial and ventricular muscular syncytia are separated by fibrous tissue that surrounds and supports the valvular rings. If one atrial fiber becomes stimulated to depolarize, the impulse will spread and depolarize all the atrial fibers, provided they are in a repolarized state. If the conduction system is intact, the impulse will spread throughout the A-V node and continue on to depolarize the ventricles. As in the case of the atrial fibers, if one ventricular muscle cell

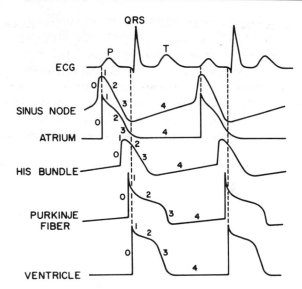

Figure 1–8 ▪ Action potentials for the sinus node, atrium, His bundle, Purkinje fibers, and ventricular myocardium are shown relative to the production of the surface ECG. The corresponding phases of each action potential are labeled, representing electrolyte shifts across the cell membrane (see text). Note the difference in action potential shape, particularly the slope of phase 4 of the normal cardiac pacemaker (sinus node). (From Edwards, NJ: Bolton's Handbook of Canine and Feline Electrocardiography, ed 2. Philadelphia, WB Saunders, 1987, with permission.)

depolarizes, all the ventricular muscle cells will depolarize. This is advantageous in the production of a single, forceful contraction of the cardiac chambers. The mechanism by which these cardiac fibers become so conductive and so easily stimulated seems to originate in the region of longitudinal gap junctions. Cell membranes

ordinarily possess high internal electrical resistance, but the cardiac cell membranes in the region of the gap junctions have extremely low resistance. They are consequently easily stimulated, and the cell-to-cell transfer of electrical current in the cardiac syncytium is facilitated.

THE CARDIAC CONDUCTION SYSTEM

The cardiac conduction system is responsible for organizing the sequence of depolarization of the heart. These specialized tissues conduct electrical impulses through the heart rapidly, so that all the cardiac muscle fibers in the atrial syncytium or in the ventricular syncytium contract almost simultaneously to produce a forceful contraction. At the same time, a delay is built into the system at the A-V node to allow time for the atria to fill the ventricles actively before ventricular contraction occurs. The conduction system consists of the S-A node, the interatrial bundles, the A-V node, the common bundle of His, the right and left branches of the bundle of His, and the Purkinje fibers (see Fig. 1–3).

The Sinoatrial Node

The S-A node is a small strip of specialized cardiac muscle located at the junction of the right atrium and the cranial vena cava. It is the usual cardiac pacemaker because it has the most rapid rate of automatic or spontaneous discharge; its cells have the most rapid rate of inward Na^+ movement through the cell membrane during diastolic depolarization (phase 4 of the action potential). The fibers in the S-A node have a relatively low resting transmembrane potential (Fig. 1–8).

Atrial Conduction

Once the S-A node has initiated depolarization, the electrical impulse spreads across the atria to the A-V node, producing a P wave on the ECG (Fig. 1–9A). The P wave represents the sum of all the electrical forces produced during the depolarization of both atria. Be-

cause the S-A node is located in the right atrium, the right atrium begins to depolarize about 0.01 sec before the left atrium. The P wave, thus, is a recording of first the right and then, 0.01 sec later, the left atrial depolarization (Fig. 1–10). This will become important later when atrial enlargement patterns are discussed.

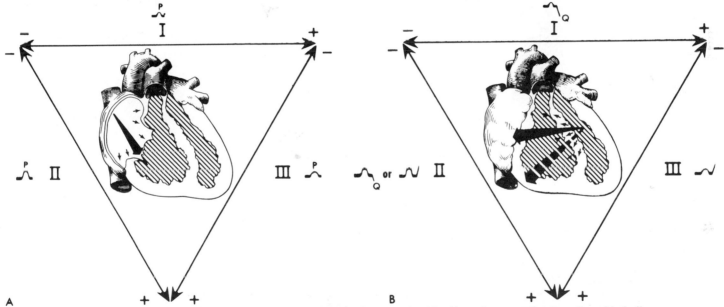

Figure 1–9 ■ *A*, After the S-A node initiates depolarization, an electrical impulse speeds across the atria to the A-V node, producing the P wave on the electrocardiogram. Leads I, II, and III form an equilateral triangle around the heart, and each lead "sees" the impulse from a different position. After the P wave occurs, the recording returns to the baseline as the P-R segment, indicating the delay in the A-V node just before the ventricles discharge. *B*, The first phase of the ventricular activation process is depolarization of the ventricular septum. This produces the Q wave or is incorporated into the R wave on the electrocardiogram. The Q wave is usually a rather small negative deflection that does not appear consistently on every normal lead II electrocardiogram. Again, each lead "sees" the impulse from its own position. (From Edwards, NJ: Bolton's Handbook of Canine and Feline Electrocardiography, ed 2. Philadelphia, WB Saunders, 1987, with permission.)

Figure continued on following page

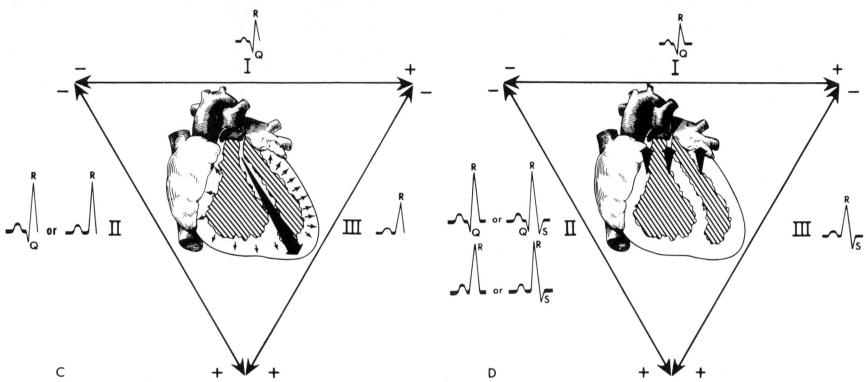

Figure 1–9 ■ *Continued C*, The second phase of ventricular activation is depolarization of the left and right ventricular free walls. This produces the R wave on the electrocardiogram, and is the largest force produced. *D*, The third and last phase of ventricular activation is depolarization of the base of the septum and both ventricles. This produces the S wave on the electrocardiogram. The S wave also occurs variably on the lead II electrocardiogram, and the four possible normal lead II tracings are shown. (*C* and *D*, adapted from Netter, FH and Yonkman, FF: The CIBA Collection of Medical Illustrations, Vol 5. Copyright by CIBA Pharmaceutical Company, Division of CIBA-GEIGY Corporation, 1969, pp. 52–53. All rights reserved.)

right A-V valve. It is composed of specialized tissue very similar to that of the S-A node. As the atrial impulse enters the node, conduction velocity slows to 100 mm/sec, preventing the impulse from entering the ventricles too soon. This allows the atria time to discharge their complement of blood into the ventricles before ventricular contraction occurs. The delay at the A-V node is recorded electrocardiographically as a straight line (isoelectric period) following the P wave, and is called the P-R *segment* (Fig. 1–12). The total amount of time required for both atrial depolarization and the delay in the A-V node is measured as the P-R *interval* (Fig. 1–12).

The A-V node is composed of three sections: the upper or junctional zone, which receives atrial input; the middle or enclosed nodal compartment, which is isolated from the atrial myocardium; and a lower zone of longitudinally oriented fibers, which penetrates the bundle of His. There is considerable ultrastructural species variation, but most have this sequential architecture. The A-V node resem-

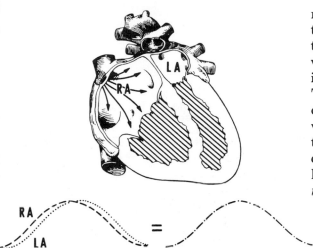

Figure 1–10 ▪ The P wave on the ECG represents the depolarization of first the right and, 0.01 sec later, the left atrium. The normal P wave, then, presents a summation of both the right and left atrial depolarization forces. This will be important in the discussion about atrial enlargement patterns. (From Edwards, NJ: Bolton's Handbook of Canine and Feline Electrocardiography, ed 2. Philadelphia, WB Saunders, 1987, with permission.)

The conduction pathways in the atria are mainly muscle to muscle, but there are also three interatrial conduction bundles that run more directly from the S-A node to the A-V node via the right and left atria (Fig. 1–11). The speed of impulse transmission through the atria is 500 to 1000 mm/sec.

The Atrioventricular Node

The A-V node lies in the septal wall of the right atrium, craniodorsal to the septal cusp of the

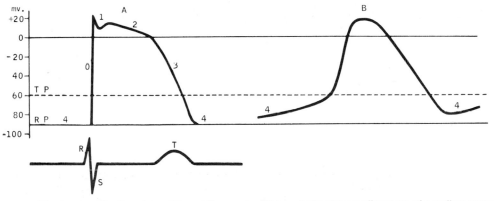

Figure 1–11 ▪ Diagrammatic drawing of the action potential and electrocardiogram of cardiac muscle fiber (*A*) and depolarization and action potential of pacemaker fiber (*B*) are shown. RP, resting membrane potential; TP, threshold potential at which the pacemaker spontaneously fires. 0, rapid depolarization with positive overshoot (intrinsic deflection of R wave); 1, initial return of the membrane potential toward zero; 2, plateau; 3, T wave; and 4, diastole during which pacemaker undergoes spontaneous slow depolarization until it reaches TP and fires. (The 0 on the ventrical mV scale and the 0 on the action potential A are not the same—mV 0 means the horizontal line is neither positive nor negative; phase 0 describes the initial event of the action potential.) (From Ettinger, SJ: Textbook of Veterinary Internal Medicine: Diseases of the Dog and Cat, ed 3. Vol 1. Philadelphia, WB Saunders, 1989, with permission.)

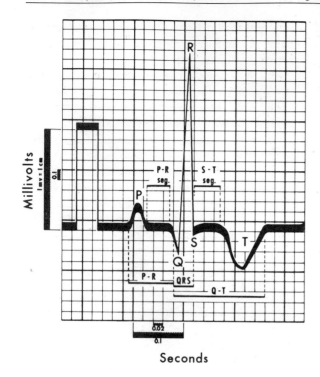

Millivolts

Seconds

Figure 1–12 ▪ A normal lead II electrocardiographic complex is shown. The electrocardiograph has been standardized at 1 cm = 1 mv, so that each small box on the vertical axis equals 0.1 mv. This tracing was recorded at 50 mm/sec paper speed, so each small box on the horizontal axis equals 0.02 sec.

Atrial depolarization is indicated by the P wave. Following the P wave, there is a short delay in the A-V node (P-R segment), after which the ventricles depolarize and produce the QRS complex. The S-T segment and the T wave represent ventricular repolarization.

Measurement of the waves in this lead II complex yields important information (see Chapter 6). The height and width of the P wave are measured. The P-R interval is measured from the beginning of the P wave to the beginning of the QRS complex. The width of the QRS complex and the height of the R wave from the baseline up are measured. The S-T segment should return to the baseline for a short time before slipping into the T wave, as it does here. The Q-T interval is measured from the beginning of the QRS complex to the end of the T wave.

The measurements for this complex are as follows:

P = 0.04 sec (2 boxes) by 0.2 mv (2 boxes)
P-R interval = 0.09 sec (4-1/2 boxes)
QRS width = 0.05 sec (2-1/2 boxes) by R wave of 1.7 mv (17 boxes)
S-T segment and T wave = normal
Q-T interval = 0.18 sec (9 boxes)

(From Edwards, NJ: Bolton's Handbook of Canine and Feline Electrocardiography, ed 2. Philadelphia, WB Saunders, 1987, with permission.)

bles a sponge somewhat, with the holes representing specialized conduction pathways through a fibrous nodule. Extensive cholinergic and adrenergic fiber innervation also occurs in this region.

The Bundle of His and Purkinje System

The bundle of His leaves the A-V node and courses into the ventricular septum, where it divides into the right and left bundle branches. The bundle branches run just beneath the septal endocardium. The right bundle travels down the right side of the ventricular septum and supplies the right ventricle through a network of conducting fibers. The left bundle travels down the left side of the ventricular septum, divides into anterior and posterior fascicles, and continues along the septum toward the apex as the septal fascicle. The Purkinje fibers are the terminations of the bundle branches in the walls of the ventricles. In the dog, cat, and ferret the Purkinje fibers terminate subendocardially, whereas in the horse and cow they extend deeper into the myocardium. Conduction through this portion of the system is rapid (2000 mm/sec), so that the entire ventricular muscle mass contracts synchronously to produce a forceful beat.

There are three main phases in the usual sequence of ventricular depolarization. These three phases, or waves of electrical activity, produce the Q, R, and S deflections on the ECG. The Q wave is the first negative (downward) deflection on the lead II ECG. It represents the first phase of the ventricular depolarization and is produced by the discharge of the middle and apical portions of the ventricular septum (Fig. 1–9B). The electrical impulses spread from the left septal surface toward the right, and from the right septal surface toward the left. The ECG records them as left-to-right and caudal-to-cranial forces because these impulses are of so much greater magnitude that they override the right-to-left forces. The second vector then becomes the return to the baseline, or the isopotential point.

The R wave is the first positive (upward) deflection on the lead II ECG. It is produced during the next phase of ventricular depolarization and is normally the greatest force produced (Fig. 1–9C). It occurs as the impulse spreads from the terminations of the Purkinje system toward the epicardial surfaces of both ventricles, via conduction from muscle fibers in the ventricular free walls. Even though both the left and right ventricles discharge simultaneously, the ECG records the deflection as if only the left ventricular forces were present. This occurs because the left ventricular forces are of much greater magnitude and usually cancel out the smaller right ventricular electrical forces.

The third phase of the ventricular depolarization produces the S wave, which is the first negative (downward) deflection that occurs following the R wave on the lead II ECG. This deflection occurs as the muscle fibers at the base of the heart are activated in an apicobasilar direction (Fig. 1–9D).

Thus, although many electrical forces are produced, three major waves of electrical activity are usually recorded during ventricular depolarization on the ECG. The Q wave in lead II represents septal activation, the R wave in lead II indicateas ventricular free wall myocardial activation, and the S wave in lead II signifies depolarization of the basal septal and ventricular basilar portions of the heart. The direction of the main force (the R wave) varies only slightly, but the Q and S waves are usually quite small deflections that do not appear consistently in every normal ECG. There are several normal variations of the QRS configurations that may occur (Fig. 1–13). The different leads record a different view of this sequence, as though the object were being observed from several different angles.

INNERVATION OF THE HEART

The heart is generously supplied with both sympathetic and parasympathetic nerves that regulate heart rate, conduction of electrical impulses, and contractility of the myocardium. Cardiac nerves may contain sympathetic or parasympathetic fibers, or both. The left and right ansa subclavia, the ventrolateral cardiac nerve, and the right stellate cardiac nerve are mainly sympathetic in action. The right thoracic vagus is predominantly parasympathetic in origin. The left thoracic vagus, ventromedial, craniovagal, and right recurrent cardiac nerves all contain both sympathetic and parasympathetic fibers. In general, however, para-

sympathetic nerves are distributed mainly to the S-A node, the atrial myocardium, the A-V node, and the most proximal portion of the ventricular conduction system, whereas the sympathetic nerves are distributed mainly to the A-V node and ventricular myocardium (Fig. 1–14). Some sympathetic fibers do terminate in the S-A node and atrial myocardium. Generally, the right sympathetic trunk supplies the right atria and ventricle, whereas the left sympathetic trunk supplies the left ventricular myocardium.

Stimulation of the vagus nerves increases parasympathetic tone, which decreases the heart rate and slows conduction through the A-V node. Excessive vagal activity can completely stop the rhythmicity of the S-A node or completely block impulse transmission through the A-V node. These vagal effects are mediated by the release of acetylcholine, which increases cell membrane permeability to K^+. The cells lose K^+, which increases intracellular negativity, the cells are then said to be hyperpolarized, so that far greater quantities of Na^+ must enter the cells to attain the threshold potential and stimulate depolarization. Parasympathetic tone is influenced by respiratory activity, ocular pressure, intracardiac and intrapulmonary receptors, and stimulation of the carotid sinus. Variation in parasympathetic tone will cause cardiac rate and rhythm to change. This so-called sinus arrhythmia, which is mediated through the vagus nerve, is normal for the dog and horse. Certain respiratory diseases may accentuate this phenomenon. In the cat, however, vagal tone has much

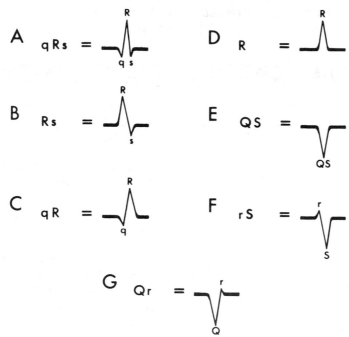

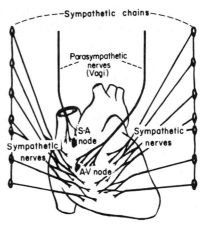

Figure 1–14 ■ The cardiac nerves. (From Guyton, AC: Textbook of Medical Physiology, ed 7. Philadelphia, WB Saunders, 1986, with permission.)

Figure 1–13 ■ By definition, the Q wave is the first negative (downward) deflection on the electrocardiogram. The R wave is the first positive (upward) deflection, and the S wave is the first negative deflection following the R wave. This must be kept in mind when determining whether there is a Q, R, or S wave present. For labeling purposes, the major deflection is indicated by a capital letter and the minor deflections by lower case letters. When discussing QRS morphology, it is important to describe the waves in this manner. A, This complex has all three deflections: a small negative q, a large positive R, and a small s wave. B, There is no Q wave in this complex; a small s wave follows the large positive R wave. C, There is no S wave in this complex; the small q wave precedes the large positive R wave. D, The S and Q waves are missing in this complex, with only the R wave present. E, When only a negative wave is present, as in this instance, it is considered that both the Q and S waves are present. F, There is no Q wave in this abnormal complex; instead, a small r wave precedes a large S wave. G, There is no S wave in this abnormal complex; a large Q wave precedes the small r wave. The first four complexes (A, B, C, and D) are normal variations of the lead II electrocardiogram (see Fig. 1–9D). (From Edwards, NJ: Bolton's Handbook of Canine and Feline Electrocardiography, ed 2. Philadelphia, WB Saunders, 1987, with permission.)

less influence on the S-A node and consequently sinus arrhythmia is not usually seen in this species unless some disease state exists.

Stimulation of the sympathetic nerves causes an increase in the rate and force of contraction; it is mediated by the release of norepinephrine at the nerve endings. Norepinephrine may increase the permeability of the cell membranes to both Na^+ and Ca^{2+}. The rapid entrance of Na^+ into the cells causes the threshold potential to be reached quickly and depolarization to occur more rapidly. The increased availability of Ca^{2+} may be responsible for the increased force of contraction.

Sensory receptors have vagal afferent pathways present within the left ventricular wall.

Stimulation of these inhibitory cardiac receptors by stretch, chemical substances, or drugs increases parasympathetic activity and decreases sympathetic activity, causing reflex bradycardia, vasodilation, and hypotension (Bezold-Jarisch reflex). These receptors also modulate renin and vasopressin activity. Decreases in the activity of this receptor system reflexly increase sympathetic tone, vasoconstriction, and plasma renin and vasopressin activity. In addition, emotional stimulation and exercise result in an increase in circulating epinephrine of adrenal origin, which has sympathetic actions on the heart similar to those of norepinephrine.

Key Words Review

Automaticity Property that allows a cell to reach its threshold potential spontaneously owing to slow inward movement of Na^+ ions.

Conductivity Property that allows electrical current to travel from one part of the heart to another.

Excitability Property that describes the ease with which a cell can become depolarized.

Dysrhythmia An abnormal, usually irregular heart rhythm, generally originating from outside the normal pacemaker area.

Electrocardiogram A sequence of atrial and ventricular depolarizations and repolarizations, depicted on a monitor screen or paper tracing.

Electrocardiograph The machine that records the electrocardiogram.

Amplitude The height of any given waveform of the ECG, which corresponds to the amount of electrical activity sensed by the electrode.

Duration The width of any given waveform of the ECG, which corresponds to the duration of time electrical activity is being sensed by the electrodes.

P Wave The first wave of the normal ECG sequence and represents the sum of all electrical forces produced during depolarization of both atria.

QRS Complex Made up of the Q wave, R wave, and S wave, follows the P-R segment and represents the sum of all electrical forces produced during depolarization of both ventricles.

T Wave Follows the S-T segment and represents the sum of all the electrical forces generated during repolarization of both ventricles.

P-R Interval Represents the period of time from the beginning of atrial depolarization to the beginning of ventricular depolarization.

S-T Segment Lies between the QRS and T waves and represents the period of time between the completion of ventricular depolarization and the beginning of ventricular repolarization.

Q-T Interval Measured from the beginning of the QRS complex to the end of the T wave representing the time period during which ventricular depolarization and repolarization occur.

Resting Transmembrane Potential The baseline state of an unstimulated cell as determined by the relative difference between the charges on either side of the cell membrane. It is usually −90 mv in a normal myocardial cell.

Threshold Potential The critical level to which the resting transmembrane potential must be raised to stimulate a response or generate an impulse.

Depolarization The discharge and generation of current that is produced by a cell following the inward transmembrane movement of positive ions subsequent to an electrical stimulus.

Repolarization The return of the depolarized cell to its resting state subsequent to an outward movement of positive ions.

Action Potential A rapid sequence of changes in the electrical potential across the cell membrane consisting of five phases: 0, 1, 2, 3, 4. Phases 0 through 3 compose electrical systole, and phase 4, electrical diastole. Together they represent the electrical cardiac cycle of depolarization and repolarization.

S-A Node The sinoatrial node that is composed of special cells with fast rates of spontaneous depolarization such that it is the normal cardiac pacemaker (controls the pace or rate of the heart).

A-V Node The atrioventricular node that slows atrial impulses as they enter the ventricle allowing time for the atria to finish emptying their blood into the ventricle prior to ventricular depolarization.

Purkinje System The terminal ramification of the interventricular conduction fibers. They end at various levels within the myo-cardium (heart muscle) depending on the species.

Bundle of His The portion of the specialized conduction system that connects the A-V node to the bundle branches.

Bundle Branches The right and left portions of the intraventricular conduction system, which terminates as the Purkinje system.

Sympathetic Nervous Innervation Cardiac nerve endings that are primarily distributed to the A-V node and ventricular myocardium and are responsible for increasing heart rate and force of contraction owing to release of norepinephrine.

Parasympathetic Nervous Innervation Cardiac nerve endings that are primarily distributed to the S-A node, atrial myocardium, and A-V node and are responsible for slowing the heart rate and decreasing conduction through the A-V node because of release of acetylcholine.

Cardiac Conduction System All the specialized tissues of the heart that are responsible for the generation and conduction of the normal electrical impulse. Its parts include the S-A node, interatrial tracts, A-V node, bundle of His, bundle branches, and Purkinje system.

References

Edwards, NJ: Bolton's Handbook of Canine and Feline Electrocardiography, ed 2. Philadelphia, WB Saunders, 1987.

Ettinger, SJ: Textbook of Veterinary Internal Medicine — Diseases of the Dog and Cat, ed 2. Philadelphia, WB Saunders, 1983.

Ettinger, SJ, and Suter, PF: Canine Cardiology. Philadelphia, WB Saunders, 1970.

Guyton, AC: Textbook of Medical Physiology, ed 6. Philadelphia, WB Saunders, 1981.

Smith, LH, Jr, and Their, SO: Pathophysiology. The Biological Principles of Disease. Philadelphia, WB Saunders, 1981.

Zipes, DP, and Jalife, J: Cardiac Electrophysiology from Cell to Bedside. Philadelphia, WB Saunders, 1990.

CHAPTER

2

Types of Electrocardiographic Equipment

SINGLE-CHANNEL RECORDERS (Fig. 2-1)

This type of electrocardiographic (ECG) machine has one stylus and consequently records one lead at a time. Each of the limb leads (I, II, III, aVR, aVL, and aVF) and each of the chest leads are recorded consecutively on one long strip of ECG paper. The operator can control the length of each lead being recorded when using the machine in the manual mode. Some single-channel ECG machines provide an added feature of automatic lead selection whereby a preset time period of each lead will be recorded. In advanced single-channel units, a computer-based ECG analyzer is built into the unit complete with liquid crystal display (LCD) screen and printout providing ECG waveforms, measurements, heart rate analysis, and clinical comments (Fig. 2-2). Some single-channel units have internal rechargeable battery packs facilitating use where an alternate current (AC) electrical source is unavailable. Almost all single-channel ECG units are lightweight and easily portable, able to be mounted in a fixed location or mobile cart as desired. Currently single-channel ECG machines are the most common type used in veterinary medicine.

MULTIPLE-CHANNEL RECORDERS (Figs. 2-3, 2-4)

This type of ECG machine has more than one stylus (usually three) and will provide simultaneous tracings of three leads. These are usually grouped as I, II, III; aVR, aVL, aVF; V_1, V_2, V_3; and V_4, V_5, V_6. Most units provide a rhythm strip consisting of leads I, II, and III, which can be automatically or manually recorded. The V lead nomenclature used in human electrocardiography is comparable to veterinary terminology as follows:

V_1 equivalent to rV_2 (CV_5RL)
V_2 equivalent to V_2 (CV_6LL)
V_4 equivalent to V_4 (CV_6LU)
V_6 equivalent to V_{10} (V_{10})

Leads V_3 and V_5 represent lead placements anatomically between V_2 and V_4 and between V_4 and V_{10}, respectively. They receive very little attention in veterinary medicine.

Some multiple-channel ECG machines are available with a monitor screen for added ease in viewing the ECG tracing. Multiple-channel ECG machines are usually somewhat less portable than single-channel units. They do have the decided advantage, however, of being able to "see" more than one viewpoint of electrical activity at a given instant, which is often helpful in dysrhythmia detection. An additional advantage is the convenient format of recording, which facilitates storage and retrieval of ECG data.

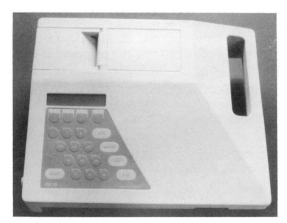

Figure 2-1 ▪ Single-channel ECG machine. (Courtesy of Seimens Burdick, Inc., Schaumburg, IL.)

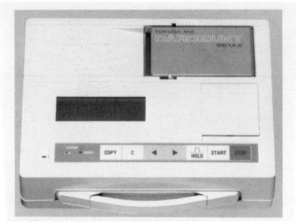

Figure 2-2 ▪ Single-channel ECG analyzer. (Courtesy of Fukuda Medical Electronics, MDICL, Inc., Weston, Ontario, Canada.)

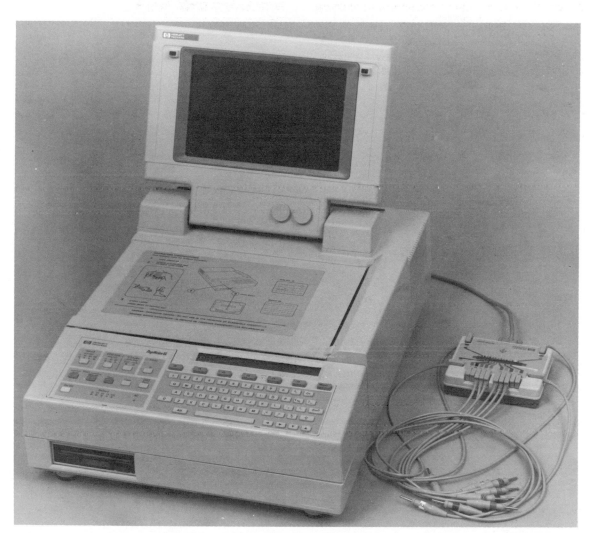

Figure 2-3 ▪ Multiple-channel ECG machine. (Courtesy of Hewlett-Packard Company, Rockville, MD.)

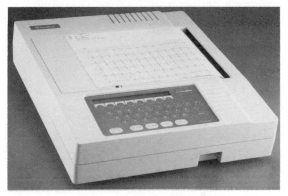

Figure 2-4 ▪ Multiple-channel ECG machine. (Courtesy of Seimens Burdick, Inc., Schaumburg, IL.)

MONITORS (Figs. 2-5, 2-6)

Oscilloscopic display or LCD monitoring of the ECG is primarily used for longer-term evaluation of the patient's heart rate and rhythm. Precise measurements of amplitude and duration of the waveforms are not easily performed utilizing the monitor format. All monitors display a continuous ECG tracing as it rolls across the screen for as long as the monitor is connected to the patient. Either single- or multiple-channel (lead) monitoring equipment is available, and most monitors can be "frozen" (stopped in place) for closer inspection of the waveforms. Many monitors have the added ability of providing a hard-copy printout of a particular ECG section of interest through an

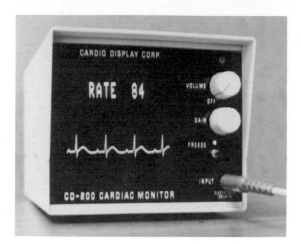

Figure 2–5 ▪ Single-channel and heart rate monitor. (Courtesy of Cardio Display Corporation, Mineola, NY.)

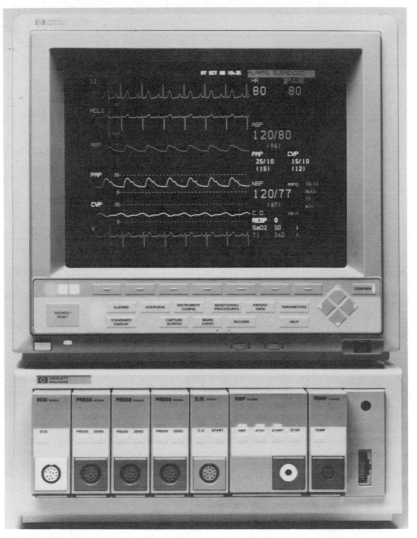

Figure 2–6 ▪ Multiple-channel monitor with ability to monitor multiple physiologic parameters, including the ECG. (Courtesy of Hewlett-Packard Company, Medical Products Group, Andover, MA.)

internalized printer or of connecting the monitor to an external ECG paper drive.

There is a wide degree of sophistication in monitoring equipment. The simplest type in veterinary medicine senses the voltage of each R wave and emits an audible signal beep without actually displaying the P-QRS-T sequence. More sophisticated units have multiple-channel capabilities for recording simultaneous ECG and blood pressure tracings, respiratory patterns, central venous pressure, and body temperature complete with preset safety ranges that, when exceeded, automatically initiate a hard-copy record of the event and sound an alarm. Newer technologies have made sophisticated monitoring innovative, compact, and affordable for veterinary use (Fig. 2–7).

ECG monitoring capabilities are built into defibrillating units as an integral part of that equipment. The patient's "preshock" rhythm can be determined and postdefibrillatory success or failure documented as well. These units are not designed to be used in routine monitoring situations. They are, however, another utilization of ECG monitoring techniques in emergency situations (Fig. 2–8).

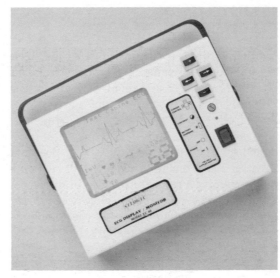

Figure 2–7 ▪ EC-60 compact, portable, multiple physiologic parameter patient monitor. (Courtesy of Silogic Electronic and Biomedical Equipment, Stewartstown, PA.)

COMPUTER ANALYZER SYSTEMS

Computer-based ECG analyzer systems are available for use with appropriately equipped IBM-compatible computers in the veterinary office. Canine and feline ECGs can be dis-

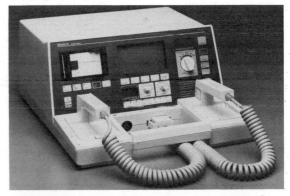

Figure 2–8 ▪ Cardiac defibrillator with ECG monitoring capability. (Courtesy of Seimens Burdick, Inc., Schaumburg, IL.)

played and integrated with diagnostic analysis programs to produce a complete ECG interpretation printout with normal reference values. The ECG tracing is immediately visible, and portions of the ECG are stored for reanalysis, if desired (Fig. 2-9).

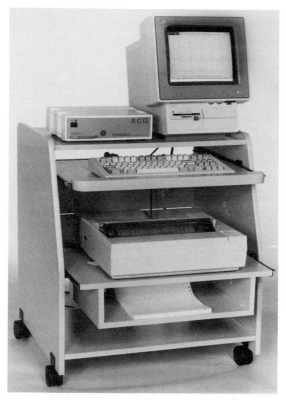

Figure 2-9 ▪ In-office ECG analyzer system. (Courtesy of Vetronics, Inc., Lafayette, IN.)

TRANSTELEPHONIC TRANSMISSION OF ECGs*

Another way to record and evaluate the ECG is to send the data transtelephonically from the veterinary office to a team of ECG specialists for analysis and interpretation. Three different ECG transmitting machines (transmitters) are available. A six-lead transmitter is designed for the veterinary office that does not have an ECG machine (Fig. 2-10). A small speaker emits a tone that varies in pitch, depending on the electrical activity of the heart. This tone is transmitted over the telephone lines to a receiver that transmits the tones into a printed ECG. A second type of transmitter (Fig. 2-11) may be used in conjunction with an ECG machine. This unit plugs into the back of most standard ECG machines and allows the technician to transmit the ECG while simultaneously running it on the ECG machine. This allows the transmitting veterinarian and the specialist to discuss the case, with both parties having a copy of the ECG to evaluate. A third unit (Fig. 2-12), a transcorder, is a battery-operated unit intended to be taken into the field, where telephones are not readily available. An ECG can be recorded and then transmitted telephonically later. All three units record six-lead ECGs (I, II, III, aVR, aVL, aVF). Patient positioning and lead placement are the same as those in recording the standard ECG (Fig. 2-13).

---

*Information for this section was provided by Dr. Francis W. K. Smith, Jr., DVM, Cardiopet, Floral Park, NY.

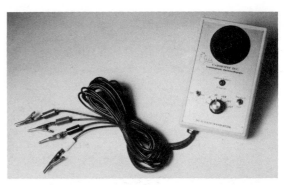

Figure 2-10 ▪ A six-lead transmitter used for transmitting ECGs transtelephonically. (Courtesy of Cardiopet, Inc., Floral Park, NY.)

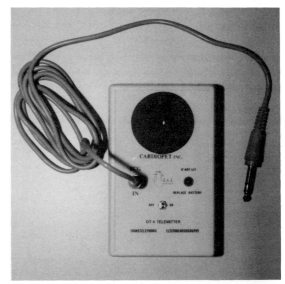

Figure 2-11 ▪ A telemitter that attaches to the back of an ECG machine for transmitting ECGs transtelephonically. (Courtesy of Cardiopet, Inc., Floral Park, NY.)

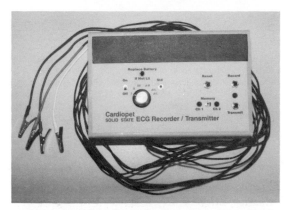

Figure 2–12 ▪ The transcorder, which allows ECGs to be recorded and transmitted transtelephonically at a later time. (Courtesy of Cardiopet, Inc., Floral Park, NY.)

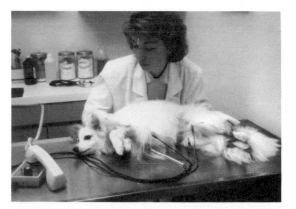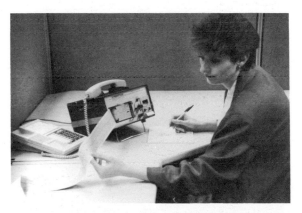

Figure 2–13 ▪ The *left panel* shows the ECG being transmitted from the veterinary office. Note that the mouthpiece of the phone is placed over the speaker on the transmitter. The *right panel* shows the ECG being received in the specialist's office. (Courtesy of Cardiopet, Inc., Floral Park, NY.)

Single-Channel Recorder An ECG machine that records one lead at a time.

Multiple-Channel Recorder An ECG machine that records more than one lead at a time.

ECG Monitor An oscilloscopic screen display or LCD of the continuous electrocardiogram.

Computer Analyzer Systems A computer system that records the patient's ECG, analyzes the waveforms, and prints out a report.

Transtelephonic Transmission A system for converting the electrical current generated by the ECG into digital tones that are transmitted via telephone lines to a receiver, which reconverts the signals to the ECG waveforms.

References

Smith, FWK: Written communication, 1992.

Technical Bulletin, Cardio Display Corp., 425 Meacham Avenue, Elmont, NY 11003.

Technical Bulletin, Hewlett Packard Co., Medical Products Division, 3000 Minuteman Road, Andover, MA 01810.

Technical Bulletin, MDICL, Inc., 175 Toryork Drive, Unit #6, Weston, Ontario, Canada M9L2Y7.

Technical Bulletin, Siemens Burdick, Inc., 915 North Plum Grove Road, Suite C, Schaumburg, IL 60173.

Technical Bulletin, Silogic Designs. Silogic Electronic and Biomedical Equipment, Stewartstown, PA 17363

Technical Bulletin, Vetronics, Inc., 330 Main Street, P.O. Box 709, Lafayette, IN 47902.

Technical Information, Cardiopet, Inc., P.O. Box 208, 51 Atlantic Avenue, Floral Park, NY 11002.

CHAPTER

3

Recording the Electrocardiogram

PATIENT POSITIONING AND RESTRAINT

The secret to success in recording a diagnostic electrocardiogram (ECG) is proper patient positioning, restraint, and lead placement. By convention, certain patient positions and lead placements have become standard in recording ECGs on domestic animals. The veterinary technician should be capable of recording an accurate ECG from the dog, cat, ferret, horse, and cow, because the majority of veterinary patients benefiting from electrocardiography come from these five species.

Body positions and lead placements for laboratory research animals, such as the monkey, rabbit, rat, and mouse, or for exotic pets, such as the hamster, gerbil, guinea pig, and avian species, can be readily performed using the limb lead techniques for the dog, cat, or ferret. Farm animals, such as the sheep, goat, pig, llama, or other cloven-hoofed species, are best recorded using the base-apex technique described for the horse and cow.

In the smaller species chemical restraint is often required to minimize movement and to facilitate proper positioning. Hypodermic needles may be clamped in the alligator clips and inserted subcutaneously if attachment of the clips directly to the skin creates too much discomfort. It is important to remember that detection of cardiac *enlargement* requires standard lead placements and patient positioning, whereas detection of cardiac *dysrhythmia* re-

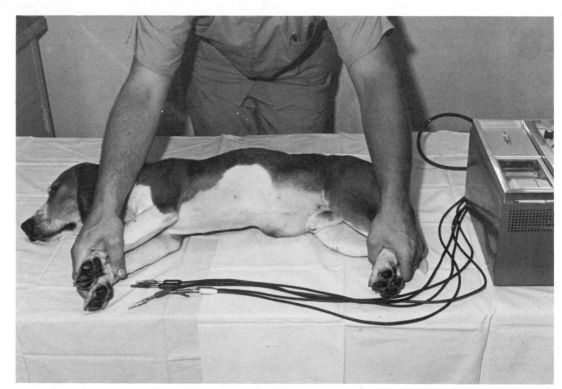

Figure 3 – 1 ▪ The conventional position used when the full electrocardiogram (ECG) is run. The dog is in right lateral recumbency. The assistant maintains the dog in this position by holding the dog's front legs with the right hand, using the right arm to hold the dog's head. The hind legs and the rump are held with the left hand and arm. The humeri and femora are held at right angles to the body and parallel to each other. The electrode cables are in position and ready to be attached to the dog. (From Edwards, NJ: Bolton's Handbook of Canine and Feline Electrocardiography, ed 2. Philadelphia, WB Saunders, 1987, with permission.)

quires only that the leads be attached to the patient regardless of lead placement or patient positioning. Whenever possible, standard patient position and lead placement should always be followed. When might standard patient positioning be unwise? If the patient is in shock, injured, or unable to stand, or if the patient would be unduly stressed if forced to assume the standard position, the ECG should be recorded in whatever position the patient is the most comfortable. This is particularly important in patients that have been hit by a car, have severe heart failure, or, in the case of large animals, may be unable to stand. Assessment of heart rhythms and measurement of waveform duration are unaffected by patient positioning or lead placement. Measurement of waveform amplitude or determination of the mean electrical axis is usually not of critical importance and can be determined later when the patient can be safely restrained in the standard position.

In the dog, cat, and ferret the standard position for ECG recording is with the patient in right lateral recumbency with the forelegs and rear legs held perpendicular to the long axis of the body and parallel to each other (Figs. 3–1, 3–2). The sternal position may be a useful alternative in the cat or ferret who resists restraint in the right lateral position (Fig. 3–3). There are minor differences seen in the waveforms in these two positions but they are usually insignificant (Fig. 3–4). The routine ECG of the horse and cow is recorded with the patient in the standing position.

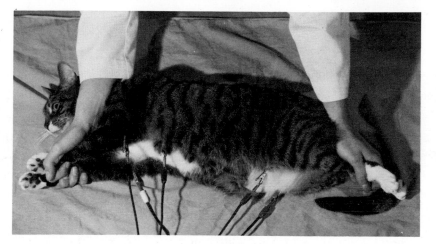

Figure 3–2 ▪ The conventional right lateral position for the feline ECG. Electrodes are shown attached just above the elbows on the forelegs and just above the stifles on the rear legs. The chest "C" electrode is shown attached at the CV_6LU (V_4) position. (From Edwards, NJ: Bolton's Handbook of Canine and Feline Electrocardiography, ed 2. Philadelphia, WB Saunders, 1987, with permission.)

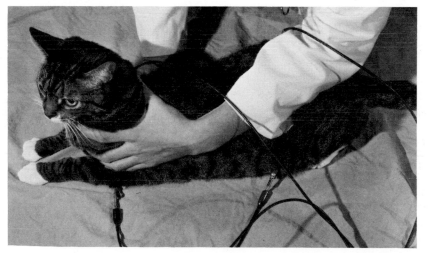

Figure 3–3 ▪ The sternal position, with the electrodes placed at the standard locations, may be used for cats or ferrets reluctant to remain quiet in the right lateral position. (From Edwards, NJ: Bolton's Handbook of Canine and Feline Electrocardiography, ed 2. Philadelphia, WB Saunders, 1987, with permission.)

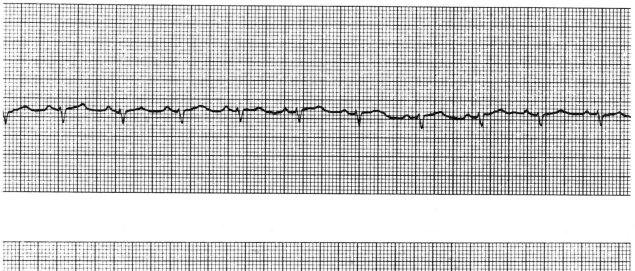

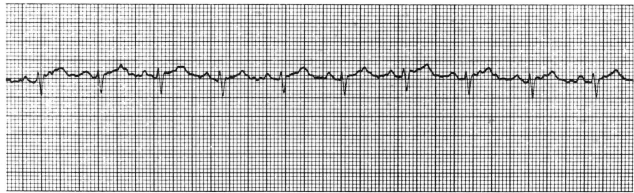

Figure 3–4 ▪ *Top*, ECG recorded from a domestic short hair cat in right lateral recumbency. 1 cm = 1 mv, paper speed 50 mm/sec. *Bottom*, ECG recorded from the same cat as in top part of this figure, this time in sternal recumbency. 1 cm = 1 mv, paper speed 50 mm/sec.

Species	Drug	Effect
Canine	Acetylpromazine 0.055 mg/kg IV	Decreases heart rate
Feline	Ketamine HCl 1.1 mg/kg IV	Increases heart rate
Ferret	Ketamine HCl 10–20 mg/kg IM and diazepam 0.25–0.5 mg/kg IM	No effect on heart rate
Equine	Zylazine 100–200 mg and butorphanol 5–7 mg IV	May slow heart rate
Bovine		
Adult cow	Zylazine 100–200 mg IV	Usually no effect on heart rate
Calf	Zylazine 5 mg IV	Usually no effect on heart rate

IV = intravenously; IM = intramuscularly.

In most instances, chemical restraint is unnecessary when recording the electrocardiogram. If chemical restraint should be necessary, the above protocols are effective without having a major influence on the ECG — with the exception of heart rate.

THE LEADS AND LEAD PLACEMENT

The leads, also called "electrodes" or "cables," are the connecting link between the patient and the ECG machine. Most single-channel ECG machines come equipped with a lead cable that encompasses five separate lead wires. Each lead wire terminates in a cylindric tip, over which No. 60 copper alligator clips, obtainable through a local hardware supplier, are placed. The end opposite the jaw end of the clip must be reshaped to fit over the end of the lead cable. This can be done with a pair of pliers or a White's small animal nail trimmer, as the clips are extremely malleable. Soldering the clips to the leads is not necessary and may actually increase the resistance to electrical conductivity as well as making removal for cleaning, repair, and replacement difficult. The teeth of the alligator clips should be filed down somewhat and the tip bent outwardly a small amount to facilitate patient comfort. In particularly thin-skinned patients cotton or a small piece of gauze sponge can be used to pad the clips.

Most oscilloscope monitors have three lead wires in the lead cable. Most multiple-channel recorders have ten lead wires. Regardless of the number of lead cables or wires the principles are the same. Figure 3–5 depicts the typical five-lead cable set used in recording the ECG with a single-channel ECG machine. A typical three-lead cable set commonly employed for oscilloscopic monitoring is shown in Figure 3–6 and a ten-lead cable set for recording with a multiple-channel ECG machine is seen in Figure 3–7. All of these lead sets are labeled (usually with human terminology) for proper placement on the patient.

The lead placement patterns can be divided into two groups — the limb leads and the chest leads. In the five-lead cable system the limb leads are labeled right arm or foreleg (RA), left arm or foreleg (LA), right rear leg (RL), and left rear leg (LL). These four lead cables record the six standard and augmented limb or frontal leads (I, II, III, and aVR, aVL, and aVF) of the electrocardiogram. The fifth lead is usually labeled C (sometimes V). This lead cable is called the exploring electrode and is moved to various positions on the patient's thorax to record the chest leads of the electrocardiogram $CV_5RL(rV_2)$, $CV_6LL(V_2)$, $CV_6LV(V_4)$, and V_{10}. These lead systems will be discussed in more detail later in this chapter. The lead cables are usually color coded as well for rapid identification: RA (white), LA (black), RL (green), LL (red), and C (brown).

The front leg leads (RA and LA) are attached to the appropriate foreleg just above the elbow. The rear leg leads (RL and LL) are likewise attached to the appropriate rear leg immediately proximal to (above) the stifle (knee) (Fig. 3–8). The exploring electrode (C lead) placements are shown in Figure 3–9, *A* and *B*. Review Figures 3–2 and 3–3 to visualize the lead placements for the cat. These same lead

Text continued on page 34

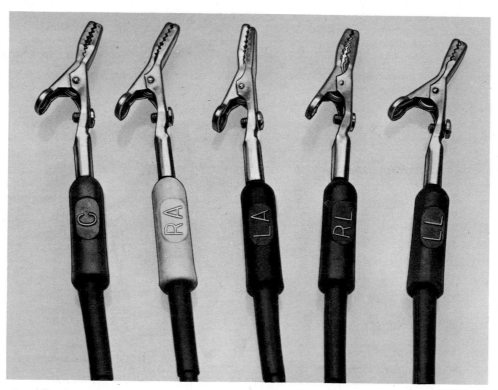

Figure 3–5 ▪ Alligator clips, no. 60 size, with the jaws bent slightly, make excellent electrodes when they are clipped to the dog's skin. The alligator clips must be securely fastened to the cable tips. (From Ettinger, SJ, and Suter, PF: Canine Cardiology. Philadelphia, WB Saunders, 1970, with permission.)

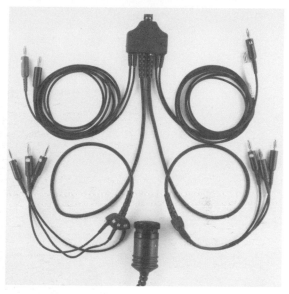

Figure 3 – 7 ▪ Patient cable and lead wire system used for recording the ECG on a multiple-channel electrocardiograph.

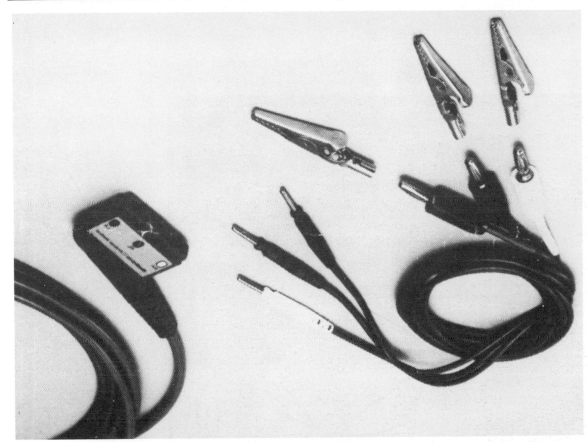

Figure 3 – 6 ▪ Modular three-lead cable systems with detachable alligator clip electrodes used for oscilloscopic monitors. (Courtesy Cardio Display Corp., Mineola, NY.)

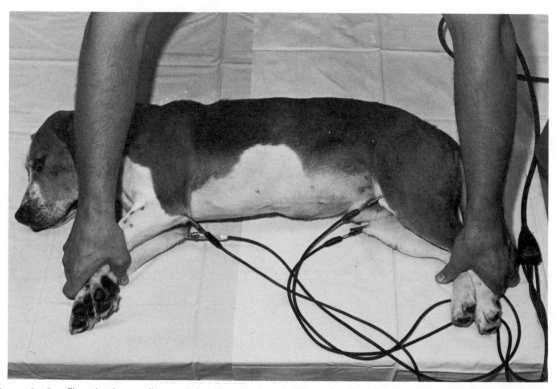

Figure 3 – 8 ▪ The electrocardiograph leads have been attached to the legs. The arm leads are placed just above the elbows, and the leg leads are placed just above the stifles. The standard six-lead electrocardiogram is run using only these four cables. The right hind leg is the ground. Note that the entire cable is placed on the table with the dog to minimize movement artifacts. (From Edwards, NJ: Bolton's Handbook of Canine and Feline Electrocardiography, ed 2. Philadelphia, WB Saunders, 1987, with permission.)

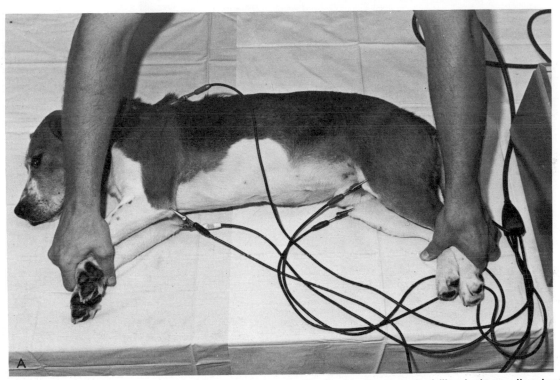

Figure 3–9 ▪ *A,* The exploring electrode in this picture is attached to the dorsal midline between the dog's scapulae, at about the seventh thoracic vertebra; this is the V_{10} exploring lead and is run on the V setting of the electrocardiograph.

Figure continued on following page

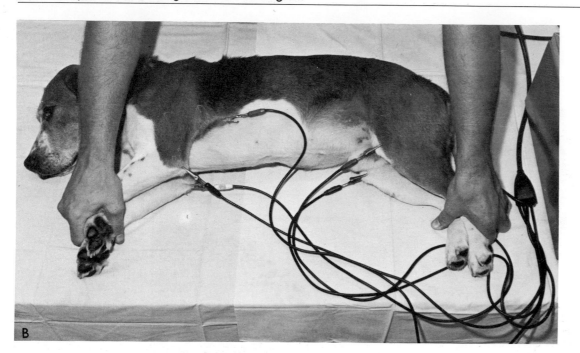

B

placements are used for the ferret. The limb lead placements for the horse can be seen in Figure 3–10 and for the cow in Figure 3–11. The base-apex electrode placement for both horse and cow is depicted in Figure 3–12.

WETTING THE CLIPS AND GROUNDING THE SYSTEM

The electrode clips should be clean and should fit tightly to the lead wires. Following placement of the clips in the proper position, the clip and skin should be moistened to establish good

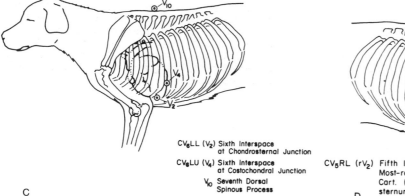

C

CV$_6$LL (V$_2$) Sixth Interspace
                at Chondrosternal Junction

CV$_6$LU (V$_4$) Sixth Interspace
                at Costochondral Junction

V$_{10}$ Seventh Dorsal
         Spinous Process

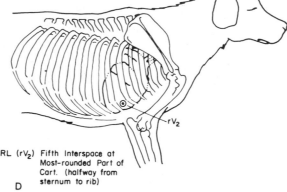

D

CV$_5$RL (rV$_2$) Fifth Interspace at
                 Most-rounded Part of
                 Cart. (halfway from
                 sternum to rib)

Figure 3–9 ▪ *Continued B,* Another exploring lead (CV$_6$LU) is produced by moving the exploring lead to a point at the left sixth intercostal space at the costochondral junction. This is also run on the V setting of the electrocardiograph. Placement positions for exploring lead (C lead) are shown, viewed from the left side (*C*) and the right side (*D*). (From Edwards, NJ: Bolton's Handbook of Canine and Feline Electrocardiography, ed 2. Philadelphia, WB Saunders, 1987, with permission.)

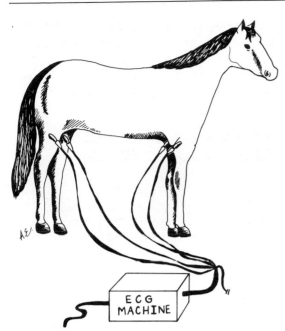

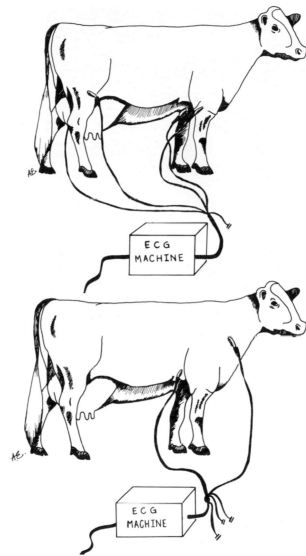

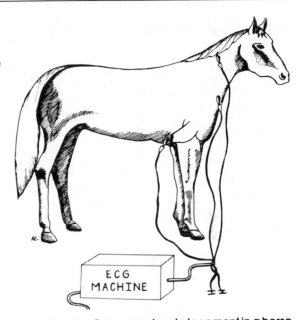

Figure 3 – 10 ▪ The limb lead placement for the horse consists of four electrodes placed as follows: Black, just above the point of the left elbow; white, just above the point of the right elbow; red, on the left stifle; green, on the right stifle. The brown electrode is not used in this lead placement system. Leads I, II, III, aVR, aVL, and aVF are recorded using this method of lead placement.

Figure 3 – 11 ▪ The limb lead placement for the cow (at top) consists of four electrodes placed as follows: Black, left elbow; white, right elbow; red, left stifle; green, right stifle. The brown electrode is left unattached. Leads I, II, III, aVR, aVL, and aVF are recorded using this system. The base apex lead system can also be used for the cow (at bottom) in the same manner as for the horse. Lead placement positions are shown.

Figure 3 – 12 ▪ Base apex lead placement in a horse is shown. The left front (black) lead is placed in the jugular furrow at the junction of the neck and body on the right side. The right front (white) lead is placed ventrally slightly to the left of the sternal midline, even with the olecranon. The right rear (green) lead is placed anywhere along the neck. The left rear (red) and central (brown) terminal are not used in this lead system. They should be taped to the lead cable so they do not touch each other and are out of the way to avoid being inadvertently stepped on by either the horse or the technician.

clip-to-skin contact (Fig. 3–13). Alcohol works well as a wetting agent and is easier to clean off the clips and hair following completion of the recording. Electrode pastes and jellies are preferred for longer-term monitoring of the ECG, as they are less likely to dry with time. Rarely is there a need to clip the hair or otherwise prepare the electrode placement sites.

Most ECG machines are equipped with either internal or external grounding wires (cables). Those units having a separate ground cable usually record best if that cable is used to connect the ECG machine to a nearby water pipe or other suitable electrical ground.

Whenever possible the ECG recording should be made with the patient on a Formica-topped table, rubber mat, foam pad, or thick blanket. This will help eliminate recording artifacts discussed in Chapter V.

Now that you have (1) reviewed the basic principles of electrocardiography, (2) become familiar with the basic types of equipment, and (3) learned how to position the patient and electrodes properly, all that remains is to familiarize yourself with the operation of the machine itself. You will then be ready to record the ECG.

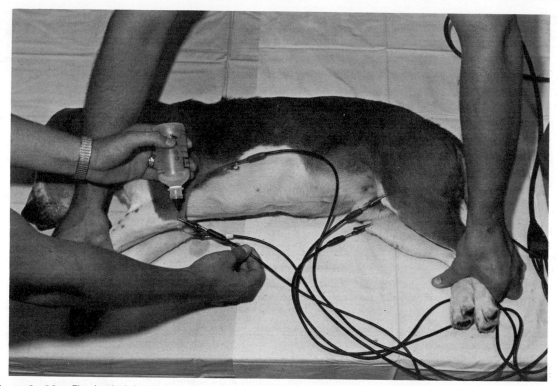

Figure 3–13 ▪ The technician is using a squirt bottle filled with alcohol to wet the electrodes and to establish good skin-to-clip contact. An assistant properly restrains the patient in right lateral recumbency. (From Edwards, NJ: Bolton's Handbook of Canine and Feline Electrocardiography, ed 2. Philadelphia, WB Saunders, 1987, with permission.)

OPERATING THE ELECTROCARDIOGRAPH

Although individual ECG machines vary widely with respect to the instrument panel array of knobs or buttons, they all have the following functions:

1. On/off switch
2. Paper speed adjustment
3. Lead selection (manual or automated)
4. Sensitivity setting
5. Standardization marker
6. Lead marking (manual or automatic)
7. Ability to maintain an "on" position without the paper drive being in motion
8. Ability to control the stylus position on the paper.

Familiarization with individual units can usually be accomplished in a short time.

Step 1. The first step should be to adjust the sensitivity control so that a 1-mv charge will deflect the stylus 1 cm. This is usually accomplished by setting the sensitivity at 1 and adjusting the standardization control accordingly. The standardization button will deliver a 1-mv charge when it is depressed (Fig. 3–14). With the sensitivity set at ½ the standard button will deflect the stylus 0.5 cm. At a sensitivity setting of 2 the standard button will deflect the stylus 2.0 cm. The ½ sensitivity setting is used when the amplitude (height) of the R wave exceeds the width of the paper, allowing the waveforms to be reduced by half in order to fit on the paper. Conversely, a sensitivity setting of 2 doubles the size of the complexes. This

can be helpful when their amplitude (height) is exceptionally small. In general all recordings should begin and end with a standardization mark of 1 (1 mv causing a stylus deflection of 1 cm) (Fig. 3–14).

Careful examination of the ECG paper (Fig. 3–15) will show a gridwork pattern divided into small 1-mm square boxes that make up larger boxes 0.5-cm square. This allows calibration of the amplitude (height) and duration (width) of the various waveforms and intervals that constitute the P-QRS-T complex. At a standard of 1, 1 cm = 1 mv; therefore, each small box equals 0.1 millivolt (mv) and each large box equals 0.5 mv of electrical activity on the vertical axis. By counting the height of the

complexes in small boxes and multiplying by 0.1, the amplitude of the complex in millivolts can be determined. It is important to remember at a sensitivity setting of ½ the height (number of small boxes on the vertical axis) must be *multiplied* by 2 to determine the millivoltage of any complex. Conversely, at a sensitivity setting of 2, height measurements must be *divided* by 2 (multiplied by 0.5) to determine the correct millivoltage.

Step 2. The paper speed adjustment should be set. Most ECG machines have variable paper speed settings at 25 mm/sec or 50 mm/sec. Some have a third paper speed of 100 mm/sec. In general the faster the expected heart rate,

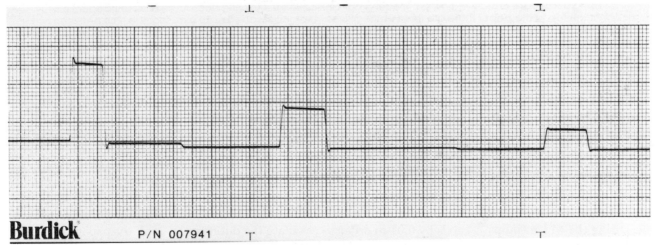

Figure 3–14 ▪ ECG strip with standard settings. The middle standard, recorded with the standard sensitivity setting of 1, shows a deflection of 10 small boxes (1 mv). The first standard was recorded with a sensitivity setting of 2 and shown a deflection of 20 small boxes (2 mv). The third standard was recorded with a sensitivity setting of ½ and shows a deflection of 5 small boxes (0.5 mv).

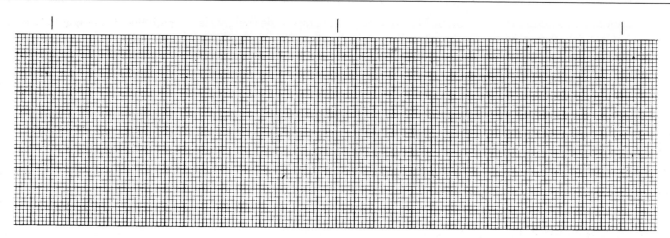

Figure 3 – 15 ▪ ECG paper with gridwork pattern allowing measurement of waveform duration (width) on a horizontal axis and waveform amplitude (height) on the vertical axis. At a paper speed of 50 mm/sec each small box along the horizontal axis equals 0.02 sec. Each large box would then equal 0.10 sec. On the vertical axis, using a standard of 1 cm = 1 mv ("I"), each small box equals 0.1 mv and each large box would equal 0.5 mv. At the top of the paper there are three vertical lines. At a paper speed of 50 mm/sec, the time between two of these lines is 1.5 sec. These vertical lines can be used to estimate the heart rate. (From Edwards, NJ: Bolton's Handbook of Canine and Feline Electrocardiography, ed 2. Philadelphia, WB Saunders, 1987, with permission.)

the faster the paper speed should be. Guidelines for initial paper speed are for the dog and cat, 50 mm/sec; ferret, 50 to 100 mm/sec; and horse and cow, 25 mm/sec.

When the ECG is recorded at a paper speed of 50 mm/sec, each small box (1 mm, 0.1 cm) on the horizontal axis represents 0.02 sec (Fig. 3 – 15). Therefore, by measuring the width (number of small boxes) of each portion of the P-QRS-T complex and multiplying by 0.02, the duration (in seconds) of electrical activity can be determined for all waveforms and intervals. When the paper speed is slowed to 25 mm/sec, each small box on the horizontal axis is multiplied by 0.04 to determine the duration (in seconds) of electrical activity. A paper speed of 100 mm/sec would require multiplication of the number of boxes on the horizontal axis by 0.01 in order to calculate the duration (in seconds) of electrical activity. At the top of the ECG paper you will find vertical marks that appear evenly spaced throughout the paper. They are used to help calculate the heart rate. At a paper speed of 50 mm/sec the time interval between two of these marks is 1.5 sec. In Chapter 6 this method of heart rate determination is explained in detail.

Step 3. Once the machine has been standardized, the paper speed selected, and the patient positioned with proper lead attachment, the paper drive is engaged and the standard button depressed once or twice. One hand should control the stylus position and the other should control the lead selector switch if it is manually operated (Fig. 3–16). When identification of the leads is not performed automatically, each lead is identified by manually depressing the marker button.

One marking system commonly used is as follows:

Lead I	-	(1 short)
Lead II	--	(2 shorts)
Lead III	---	(3 shorts)
Lead aVR	----	(4 shorts)
Lead aVL	-----	(5 shorts)
Lead aVF	------	(6 shorts)
rV_2	-----—	(5 shorts and 1 long)
V_2	-----— —	(5 shorts and 2 longs)
V_4	-----— — —	(5 shorts and 3 longs)
V_{10}	-----— — — —	(5 shorts and 4 longs).

When everything is ready the lead selector switch is placed on lead I, and the paper speed control switch on 50 mm/sec for the dog, cat, and ferret, and on 25 cm/sec for the horse and cow. One hand adjusts the stylus position so that the complexes on lead I are in the middle of the paper. Five or six good complexes of each lead are all that are necessary. Similarly, leads II, III, aVR, aVL, and aVF are recorded and marked while one hand keeps the complexes of each lead in the center of the paper. The lead

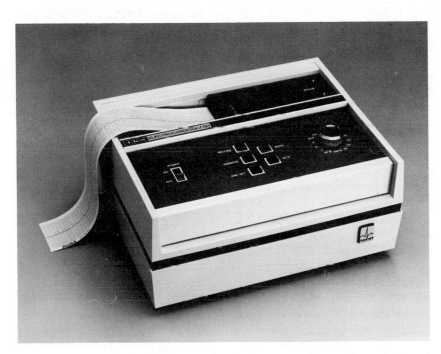

Figure 3 – 16 ▪ Control panel of a typical electrocardiograph. One hand is used to control lead selection and marking, while the other is used to maintain the stylus position in the center of the ECG paper. It is always best to use two hands when recording an electrocardiogram. (Courtesy of the Burdick Corporation, Milton, WI.)

selector switch is then returned to lead II, and 12 to 18 inches of lead II rhythm strip are recorded. If the specialized exploring leads are to be run, the C clip (brown) is attached to each designated position (see Fig. 3 – 9, *C* and *D*) and wetted. On single-channel ECG machines, all the exploring leads are run with the lead selector switch in the V lead position. Six to eight complexes are recorded and the exploring electrode is moved to its next position. This procedure is continued until all the chest lead positions have been recorded.

If the complexes are too large to fit on the paper completely, the sensitivity control switch is changed to half sensitivity. Machines that do not have this switch are restandardized so that 0.5 cm equals 1 mv. If the ECG complexes are very small, they can be doubled in size by changing the sensitivity control switch to 2 or by restandardization to 2 cm = 1 mv. These changes in sensitivity should be marked so that, when the ECG is read, the reader will remember to adjust the amplitude measurements accordingly. The duration measurements are unaffected by changes in standardization. The standard button should be pushed to record the sensitivity used at the beginning and end of each recording, or whenever a change in sensitivity is made. Multiple-channel ECG machines with ten-lead wire systems eliminate the need to move the exploring (C) electrode because the extra lead wires are already in place at their various locations on the thorax.

MONITORING TECHNIQUES

ECG monitoring usually involves continuous or intermittent evaluation of heart rate and rhythm utilizing oscilloscopic monitors with direct lead attachments to the patient, telemetry, Holter monitoring, or the ECG machine itself. Usually one to three leads are recorded, and positioning of the patient is not important. In the absence of conventional monitors the single-channel ECG machine can be used in a monitoring capacity. Lead II is usually the best lead. The machine may be left in the "on" position with the lead selector switch in the lead II position but the paper drive disengaged.

With a minimum of practice the technician can learn to use the noise of the stylus movement as an indicator of both rate and rhythm. (This will cause an accumulation of debris on the stylus tip over time, necessitating more frequent replacement of the stylus, but it can be effective when an oscilloscopic monitor is not available.) Periodically the paper drive can be engaged to obtain a representative sample of the patient's heart rate and rhythm. Usually 1 to 2 feet of a lead II rhythm strip is sufficient. Because the average heart, depending on the species, beats 30,000 to 200,000 times per day, continuous or intermittent monitoring provides a more accurate picture of heart rate and rhythm than would a relatively short ECG tracing. This becomes increasingly important if a dysrhythmia has been identified in the routine ECG; during times of shock, injury, or anesthesia; or in evaluating the patient's response to dysrhythmia therapy. ECG pastes or gels should be applied at the electrode placement site during prolonged monitoring, as they do not dry out and lose their conductivity as rapidly as does alcohol.

Telemetry is a technique of utilizing wireless transmission of the ECG tracing from a transmitter and electrodes attached to the patient's body to a monitoring screen in another location. This technique allows monitoring of more than one patient at a central monitoring station. Holter monitoring is performed by continuously recording each and every P-QRS-T complex over a 24-hour period on a tape recorder attached to electrodes placed on the patient. The tape is then processed by computer so that each complex can be evaluated.

ECG STORAGE AND RETRIEVAL

For all patients that have had an ECG, those findings should be recorded as part of their permanent medical record. In general a separate sheet containing only the ECG data is preferred to writing the ECG report in the middle of other portions of the record. Figure 3 – 17 represents one example of an ECG report. Minimum information should include patient identification, ECG identification, analysis of heart rate and rhythm, measurement of all waveforms and intervals, determinations of the mean electrical axis, ECG diagnosis, assessment, and treatment plan. Chapter 6 will cover these measurements in detail.

The ECG tracing itself may be stored directly in the medical record or either alphabetically or numerically in a separate medical record file for ECGs. Most veterinary practitioners prefer to save the entire ECG recording regardless of the method of storage, although occasionally it may be preferable to cut out representative portions of the ECG and mount them on an 8½ × 11-inch card or paper for storage. ECG paper stores well without fading, can be folded in an accordion style or rerolled in the same manner as the original ECG paper roll, and can be stored in either an envelope (folded or rolled) or a pill-dispensing vial (rolled). Placement of a rubber band around the rerolled ECG strip will facilitate storage as well. Placement of the ECG in an 8½ × 11-inch protective plastic sheet works well for direct inclusion in the folder system of medical records. Some ECG machines record short sections of multiple leads on a single sheet of 8½ × 11-inch paper, which can be readily incorporated into the patient's folder.

Regardless of the method used, the key to success will be the ability to retrieve the tracing at a future date. Such retrieval is facilitated by maintaining an ECG log book or computer entry sheet in which all ECGs are recorded and identified (Table 3–1).

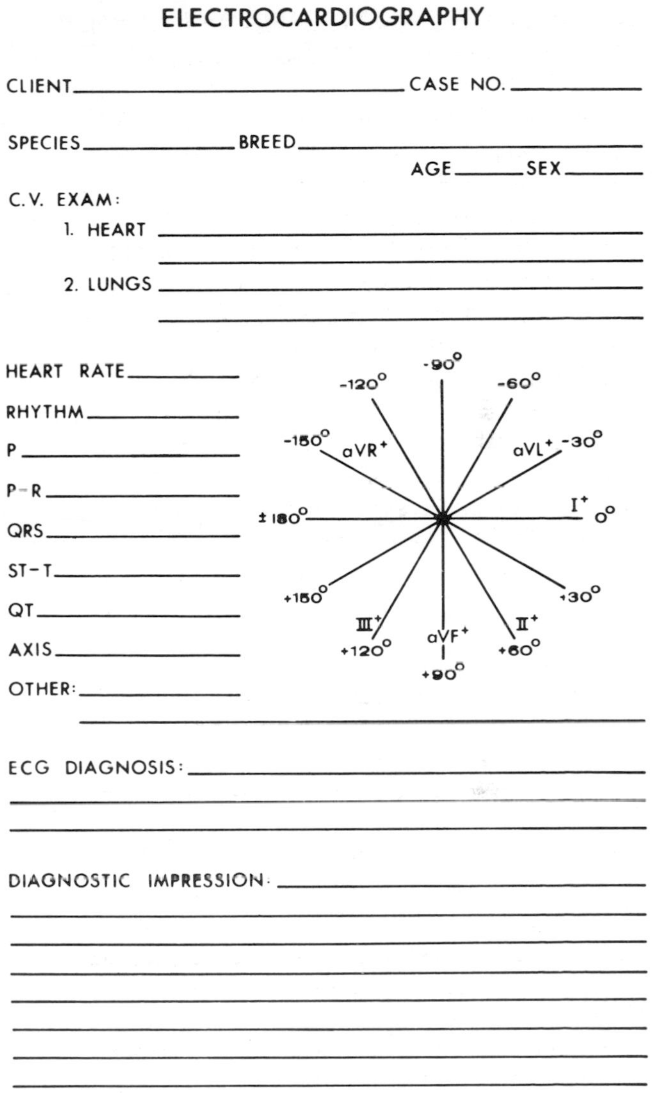

ELECTROCARDIOGRAPHY

CLIENT_____ CASE NO. _____

SPECIES_____ BREED_____

AGE_____ SEX_____

C.V. EXAM:

1. HEART _____

_____

2. LUNGS _____

HEART RATE_____

RHYTHM_____

P _____

P–R _____

QRS_____

ST–T_____

QT _____

AXIS_____

OTHER:_____

_____

ECG DIAGNOSIS:_____

_____

_____

DIAGNOSTIC IMPRESSION_____

_____

_____

_____

_____

_____

_____

_____

Figure 3–17 ▪ A form such as this one is designed for recording the ECG findings. Findings on physical examination may be recorded, and a case summary including chest x-ray findings may be written under "diagnostic impression." This form can be stored with the animal's record. (From Edwards, NJ: Bolton's Handbook of Canine and Feline Electrocardiography, ed 2. Philadelphia, WB Saunders, 1987, with permission.)

TABLE 3 – 1 ▪ Sample ECG Log

ECG No.	Date	Client	Patient	Diagnosis	Storage Location*
001	3/15/91	Edwards	"Kaitlin"	Sinus arrhythmia	Medical Records
002	3/16/91	Heber	"Angel"	Normal sinus rhythm	Medical Record No. 06729
003	3/16/91	Yohey	"Kelly"	Atrial tachycardia	Envelope No. 003
004	3/17/91	Kabrehl	"Meagan"	Ventricular tachycardia	Vial No. 004
005	3/18/91	Spring	"Fletcher"	Atrial fibrillation	Medical Records, Deceased
006	3/19/91	Peck	"Shadow"	Normal	File Cabinet No. 1(P)

*Although different locations are shown as examples, one system should be chosen and adhered to. If the medical record is placed in a separate location, such as in the case of "Fletcher" Spring, notation of that location will facilitate retrieval.

Key Words Review

Amplitude The height of any given waveform; a measurement of electrical current (voltage).

ECG Leads Recordings taken from different locations utilizing two or more electrode placements on the body. The leads are usually designated as leads I, II, III, aVR, aVL, aVF, V_1 (rV_2 or CV_5RL), V_2 (CV_6LL), V_3, V_4 (CV_6LU), V_5 and V_6 (V_{10}).

Electrodes Clips or needles that connect the patient to the lead cables.

Lead Cables Wire cables that connect the patient to the electrocardiograph.

Standard Limb Leads The recordings using any two of the electrodes on the right foreleg, left foreleg, and left rear leg; designated leads I, II, and III.

Augumented or Unipolar Limb Leads The leads that compare the positive electrode of each of the standard limb leads with the zero electrical reference point at the center of the heart; designated aVR, aVL, and aVF.

Chest Leads The recordings taken from various locations of electrode placement on the chest; also called precordial; designated V_1 (rV_2, CV_5RL), V_2 (CV_6LL), V_3, V_4 (CV_6LU), V_5 and V_6 (V_{10}).

Lead Selection Obtained by dialing the lead selector switch to the desired lead, after all electrodes have been attached to the patient.

Standardization Recording the distance the stylus travels on the vertical axis of the ECG paper when a known charge is applied to the stylus; allows measurement of the amplitude of all ECG waves by comparison to a known value.

Paper Speed Determines the measurement of the duration of waveforms and calculation of heart rate. Most ECG machines operate at paper speed of either 25 mm/sec (where one small box on the ECG paper equals 0.04 sec) or 50 mm/sec (0.02 sec per small box).

Duration The width of any given waveform, interval, or segment; a measurement of time (in seconds).

Telemetry Use of wireless transmission to transmit the ECG from the patient to a distant monitor.

Holter Monitoring A method of continuous 24-hour recording of the ECG that is stored on a tape recorder and analyzed by computer at the conclusion of the recording period.

References

Blowers, MG, and Sims, RS: How to Read an ECG, ed 4. Medical Economics Books, Oradell, NJ, 1988.

Conover, MB: Understanding Electrocardiography, ed 5. St Louis, Mosby, 1988.

Edwards, NJ: Bolton's Handbook of Canine and Feline Electrocardiography, ed 2. Philadelphia, WB Saunders, 1987.

Kelly, WJ: ECG Interpretation. Clinical Skillbuilders. Springhouse, PA, Springhouse Corp, 1990.

CHAPTER

4

Uses of the Electrocardiogram

The electrocardiogram (ECG) is an extremely valuable tool in several aspects of patient care. Table 4–1 summarizes many of these uses. The most important uses of an ECG involve the evaluation of cardiac dysrhythmias and their therapy and the monitoring of severely ill, injured, surgical, or post-surgical patients. Detection of cardiac enlargement utilizing the ECG is possible in many instances; however, the ECG is not very sensitive or specific at detecting cardiac enlargement. Usually rather significant enlargement is necessary before ECG changes can be seen. In some instances, particularly in the cat, significant enlargement (usually referred to as dilation of the heart; i.e., enlargement of the chambers) or hypertrophy (usually referred to as thickening of the heart muscle) may be present without any ECG changes (Fig. 4–1, *A, B,* and *C*). The ECG changes that occur with enlargement are discussed in detail in Chapter 6. As you would expect, dilation or hypertrophy of the atria results in enlargement of the P waves and dilation or hypertrophy of the ventricles results in enlargement of the QRS complex (Fig. 4–2).

EVALUATION OF CARDIAC DYSRHYTHMIAS

The ECG is indispensable in accurately assessing an abnormally irregular heartbeat (dysrhythmia). Irregular heartbeats are usu-

TABLE 4–1 ▪ Uses of Electrocardiography

Evaluation of Cardiac Diseases
    Evaluation of anatomic cardiac changes (cardiac enlargement)
    Evaluation of arrhythmias
    Evaluation of pericardial diseases
    Evaluation of therapy
        Drug therapy
        Electrolyte disturbances
        Pericardiocentesis
    Prognosis
    Progression of disease
    Evaluation of extracardiac diseases (e.g., pleural effusion)

Differentiation of Nonspecific Diseases that Cause Weakness, Fatigue, Lethargy, Collapse, or Seizures
    Metabolic diseases with electrolyte alterations
        Adrenal insufficiency
        Diabetic ketoacidosis
        Severe renal insufficiency
        Hypocalcemia
        Idiopathic hypokalemia
    Cardiac syncope
        Bradycardias
        Tachycardias
        Conduction disturbances
    Epilepsy
    Endocarditis, myocarditis, and cardiac neoplasia
    Systemic diseases with toxemias
    Thyroid disorders

Monitoring During Anesthesia and Surgery
    Depth of anesthesia
    Ventilation-oxygenation changes

Routine Basis
    Yearly physicals (preventive medicine)
    Evaluation prior to anesthesia and surgery
    Evaluation of trauma cases

Documentation of Data

Sharing Information and Seeking Consultation

From Edwards, NJ: Bolton's Handbook of Canine and Feline Electrocardiography, ed 2. Philadelphia, WB Saunders, 1987, p 2, with permission.

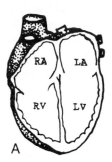 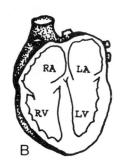 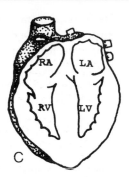

Figure 4–1 ▪ *A*, Schematic diagram shows a longitudinal section of a heart with dilated (enlarged) chambers and normal to thin muscular walls. This is referred to as cardiac dilatation. *B*, Schematically depicted normal cardiac chambers and muscular walls are shown in longitudinal section of the heart. *C*, Schematic diagram shows a longitudinal section of a heart with hypertrophy (thickening) of the muscular walls of the heart. This may occur with normal or enlarged chambers (eccentric hypertrophy) or with small chambers (concentric hypertrophy), as depicted here.

Figure 4–2 ▪ Biventricular enlargement is characterized by a wide QRS complex, tall R waves, deep Q waves. The S-T segment is usually slurred, and the P wave often indicates enlargement of one or both atria. In this lead II tracing, *A* was run at full sensitivity and *B* (same ECG) at half sensitivity. *A*, The R waves are so tall and the Q waves so deep that the tracing cannot fit on the paper. *B*, Even at half-sensitivity the complex fills the paper; the P wave is wide (0.06 sec, or three boxes) and notched (indicating P mitrale or left atrial enlargement), and the Q waves are 2.8-mv deep (double the measurement in strip B), suggesting right ventricular enlargement. Also, the R waves are too tall (6.6 mv, or 66 boxes), the QRS complexes are too wide (0.10 sec, or five boxes), and the S-T segment is slurred. All three of these abnormalities suggest left ventricular enlargement. (*A*, paper speed = 50 mm/sec, 1 cm = 1 mv; *B*, paper speed = 50 mm/sec, 0.5 cm = 1 mv.) (From Edwards, NJ: Bolton's Handbook of Canine and Feline Electrocardiography, ed 2. Philadelphia, WB Saunders, 1987, with permission.)

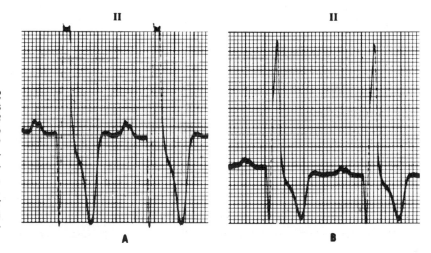

ally detected by physical examination through auscultation of the heartbeat, usually in conjunction with simultaneous palpation of a peripheral artery pulse. Logic would dictate that under normal circumstances each heartbeat should be closely followed by a pulse wave, as the blood pumped out of the heart flows through the arteries. When suddenly no pulse is present following a heartbeat heard with the stethoscope, a pulse deficit is said to be present. Pulse deficits are almost always associated with cardiac dysrhythmias. Not only does the ECG confirm the existence of the dysrhythmia but in most cases it also indicates the site of origin of the ectopic (abnormal) beat responsible for the dysrhythmia (Figs. 4–3 and 4–4). Chapter 6 discusses the recognition of abnormal rhythms in detail.

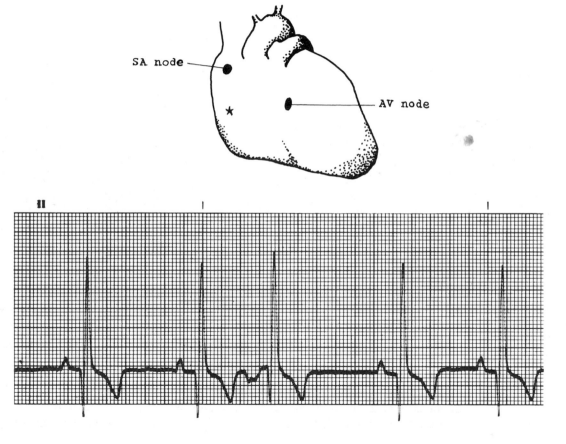

Figure 4–3 ■ This lead II ECG tracing demonstrates an abnormal complex arising from an area above the A-V node (third complex from the left). It occurs earlier than would be expected from looking at the regular rhythm, and because the heart would not have had time to fill adequately with blood before it beat again, no peripheral pulse would have been appreciated following the abnormal complex. Note that the QRS and T-wave portions of the complex appear almost identical to those of the other complexes. It is the P wave that is abnormal here, as it goes below the baseline and is therefore negative. This premature supraventricular complex is being caused by a problem in the heart muscle that lies above the A-V node. Note the asterisk on the drawing that accompanies this ECG. Paper speed = 50 mm/sec; 1 cm = 1 mv. (From Edwards, NJ: Bolton's Handbook of Canine and Feline Electrocardiography, ed 2. Philadelphia, WB Saunders, 1987, with permission.)

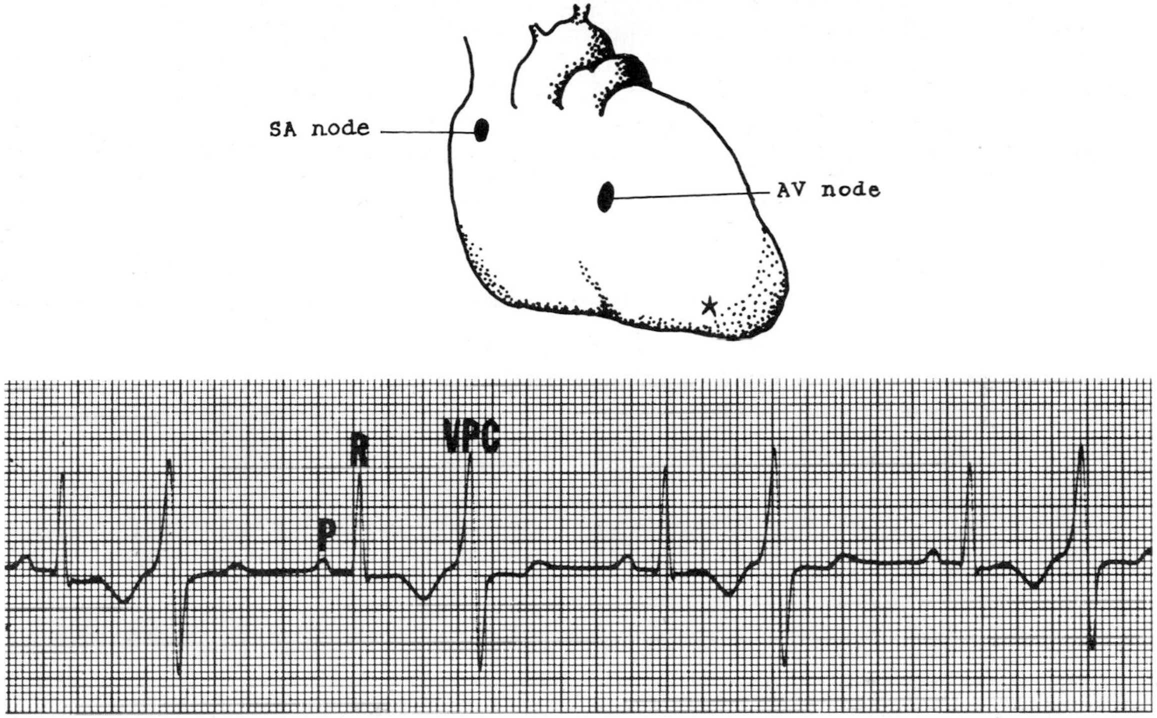

Figure 4–4 ▪ In this lead II ECG tracing, note that every other complex is abnormal and is identified here as a ventricular premature complex (VPC). The normal P-QRS-T sequence can be seen preceding each VPC. On physical examination one would hear two beats close together, but only one, in this case the first one of the pair (labeled R), would have a peripheral pulse wave associated with it. Note that the shape of the VPC is markedly different than that of the normal QRS complex. This is due to the abnormal path of conduction across the ventricle taken by the electrical current generated when the abnormal complex (VPC) was initiated. This abnormal shape confirms that the impulse did not proceed down through the bundle of His, the bundle branches, and Purkinje system, as would normally be expected, and indicates that the site of origin of the abnormal complex was below the A-V node. Consequently it is said to be of ventricular origin. Note the location of the asterisk in the drawing that accompanies this ECG. Paper speed = 50 mm/sec; 1 cm = 1 mv. (From Edwards, NJ: Bolton's Handbook of Canine and Feline Electrocardiography, ed 2. Philadelphia, WB Saunders, 1987, with permission.)

EVALUATION OF CARDIAC THERAPY

The ECG is helpful also in assessing the success or failure of therapy for cardiac disease, especially regarding those diseases that cause dysrhythmias. Frequent ECG recordings may be extremely helpful in guiding the veterinary technician and clinician in the team care of the patient receiving cardiac drugs. Administration of antidysrhythmic drugs, such as lidocaine, quinidine, procainamide, propranolol, propafenone, and the like, should normalize the rhythm, or at least improve it.

The ECG can be used to verify improvement, indicate dosage adjustment, and help to establish a prognosis based on response to therapy (Fig. 4–5). Alternatively, all antidysrhythmic drugs have the potential to make the rhythm worse following their administration, and the ECG can document this proarrhythmic effect and allow the veterinarian-technician team to switch to another drug before any serious consequences develop. Other drugs not normally considered to be antidysrhythmic drugs (potassium, calcium, digitalis glycosides, anesthetics) may have undesirable effects on

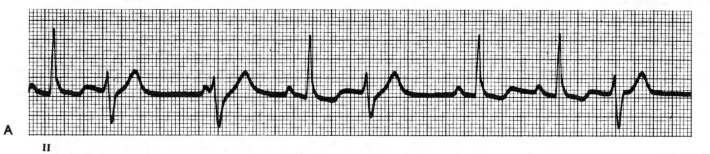

A

II

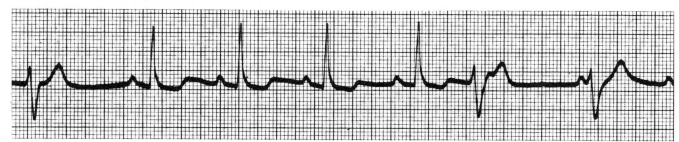

B

II

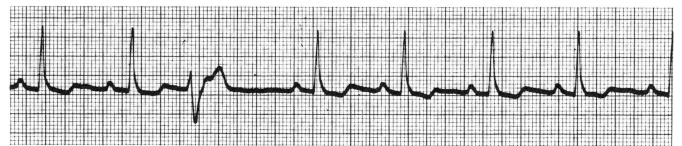

C

II

Figure 4–5 ▪ This ECG is from a 6-year-old mixed-breed dog being treated with intravenous (IV) lidocaine. *A, B,* and *C* were taken sequentially during the course of treatment. Oral quinidine was used as a maintenance medication. Note the progressive improvement in the number of VPCs during IV lidocaine therapy. Paper speed = 50 mm/sec; 0.5 cm = 1 mv. (From Edwards, NJ: Bolton's Handbook of Canine and Feline Electrocardiography, ed 2. Philadelphia, WB Saunders, 1987, with permission.)

cardiac rhythm, particularly when high levels are being administered. The ECG is helpful in guiding therapy with these agents as well (Fig. 4–6). Patients with excessively rapid or inappropriately slow heart rates may require therapy to slow down or speed up their heart rates. The ECG becomes an important tool in determining the proper dose response effect in these patients as well.

EVALUATION OF CARDIAC DISEASE PROGRESSION

Serial ECGs recorded over time provide the veterinarian-technician team the rate at which a particular disease is progressing. For example, the patient with congestive heart failure may have no dysrhythmia and little evidence of cardiac enlargement when first diagnosed. Over several months or perhaps even years, gradually progressive ECG changes may signal the need for additional therapy well before the patient's clinical signs change. Some ECG changes, particularly those occurring when patients are under stress, have recently undergone trauma, or are undergoing anesthesia, may manifest themselves over a relatively short period of time (Figs. 4–7 and 4–8). Metabolic diseases, such as adrenal insufficiency, diabetic ketoacidosis, thyroid disorders, renal disorders, portocaval shunts, hepatic cirrhosis, endotoxemia, pyometra, intestinal obstruction, pancreatitis, and septicemia, may alter myocardial electrolyte states or produce significant amounts of myocardial toxicants resulting in either dysrhythmia or mechanical dysfunction of the heart. Early

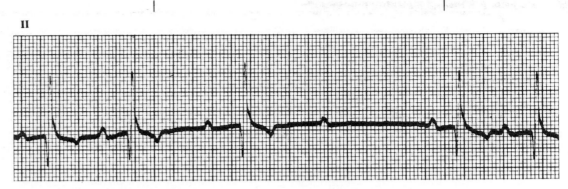

Figure 4–6 ▪ This lead II ECG was recorded from an old dog receiving digoxin. Note the progressive prolongation of the distance between the beginning of the P wave and the QRS complex (P-R interval) with a blocked P wave present following the third P-QRS-T complex. As this is an early sign of digitalis toxicity, the dosage should be reduced. (From Edwards, NJ: Bolton's Handbook of Canine and Feline Electrocardiography, ed 2. Philadelphia, WB Saunders, 1987, with permission.)

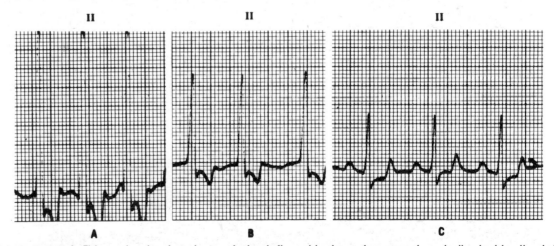

Figure 4–7 ▪ A, This canine tracing demonstrates left ventricular enlargement, as indicated by the tall R waves and the S-T segment depression. The R waves are 4.3 mv (43 boxes) tall. S-T segment depression is almost always accompanied by tall R waves or wide QRS complexes. B, This is the same dog recorded at half-sensitivity, so that the entire tracing may be placed on the paper. At half-sensitivity all height measurements must be doubled, but width measurements do not change. C, The S-T segment depression in this dog was thought to be due to hypoxia. The dog had been hit by a car and was in respiratory distress because of traumatic lung syndrome. As the lungs and the breathing improved the S-T segment changes returned to normal. (Paper speed = 50 mm/sec, 1 cm = 1 mv.) (From Edwards, NJ: Bolton's Handbook of Canine and Feline Electrocardiography, ed 2. Philadelphia, WB Saunders, 1987, with permission.)

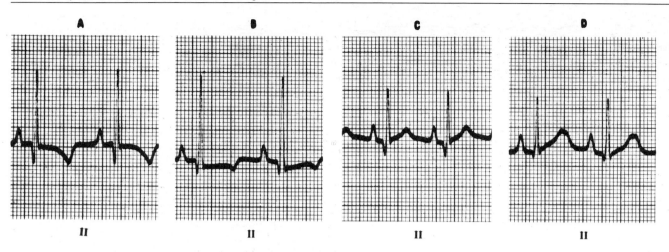

Figure 4–8 ▪ This series of electrocardiograms demonstrates the effects of myocardial hypoxia. *A*, Normal lead II tracing from a dog that is under anesthesia and is well oxygenated; *B*, This tracing shows a very early indication of myocardial hypoxia—note the change in the T-wave conformation; *C* and *D*, as the hypoxia becomes more severe, the heart rate increases slightly and the T wave actually reverses polarity and becomes positive. (From Edwards, NJ: Bolton's Handbook of Canine and Feline Electrocardiography, ed 2. Philadelphia, WB Saunders, 1987, with permission.)

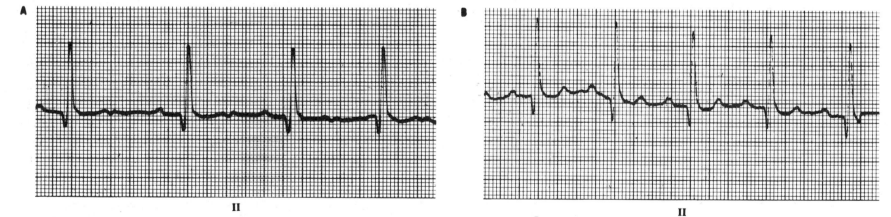

Figure 4–9 ▪ *A*, A lead II ECG recorded from a St. Bernard with hypokalemia of undetermined origin. His only clinical sign was profound weakness and inability to rise. His serum potassium level was 2.8 mEq/liter. The significant changes on the electrocardiogram were the prolongation of the Q-T interval to 0.28 sec (14 boxes) and the small biphasic T waves. *B*, Recorded after 2 days of intravenous potassium replacement therapy. The serum potassium level was 4.2 mEq/liter at the time of this recording. The dog could stand and walk with good strength. (Paper speed = 50 mm/sec, 1 cm = 1 mv.) (From Edwards, NJ: Bolton's Handbook of Canine and Feline Electrocardiography, ed 2. Philadelphia, WB Saunders, 1987, with permission.)

signs of such disorders may be seen by careful assessment of the S-T segment, T wave, or P-R segment of the ECG. Waveform changes, when noted on serial ECGs, may be the first indication of impending disaster or a dependable sign of stabilization (Fig. 4–9).

MONITORING SEVERELY ILL OR SURGICAL PATIENTS

The ECG, either by continuous monitoring (as discussed in Chapter 2) or by periodic recording of a hard copy, is a crucial part of the team management approach to the care of severely ill, traumatized, or surgical and postsurgical patients. Frequently these patients do not have or are unable to show outward signs of cardiac embarrassment even though they are present. If the veterinarian or the veterinary technician waits for symptoms to be present, it may be too late.

This is particularly true in the case of the trauma patient who may have obvious contusions, lacerations, and fractures. In these cases, one must remember that the entire body — not just the broken bone — was involved in the traumatic incident. In the assessment of the cardiovascular system of the trauma victim, the ECG is a must. All trauma patients should receive an ECG as soon as possible after the initial evaluation and triage have been completed. If any ECG abnormalities are detected, regular frequent monitoring throughout the hospitalization period is extremely important. In very severe trauma cases, dys-

rhythmias may be present on entry. However, many cases of myocardial bruising do not result in significant dysrhythmias until 12 to 96 hours after the incident. In this case, repetitive monitoring is crucial, as it is usually during this time period that most surgical corrections are performed. If dysrhythmias are not recognized and treated before anesthesia and surgery, the risks for complication and death skyrocket (Fig. 4–10).

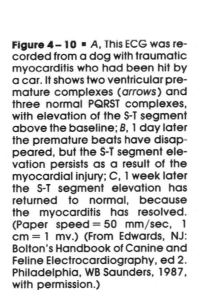

Figure 4–10 ▪ *A*, This ECG was recorded from a dog with traumatic myocarditis who had been hit by a car. It shows two ventricular premature complexes (*arrows*) and three normal PQRST complexes, with elevation of the S-T segment above the baseline; *B*, 1 day later the premature beats have disappeared, but the S-T segment elevation persists as a result of the myocardial injury; *C*, 1 week later the S-T segment elevation has returned to normal, because the myocarditis has resolved. (Paper speed = 50 mm/sec, 1 cm = 1 mv.) (From Edwards, NJ: Bolton's Handbook of Canine and Feline Electrocardiography, ed 2. Philadelphia, WB Saunders, 1987, with permission.)

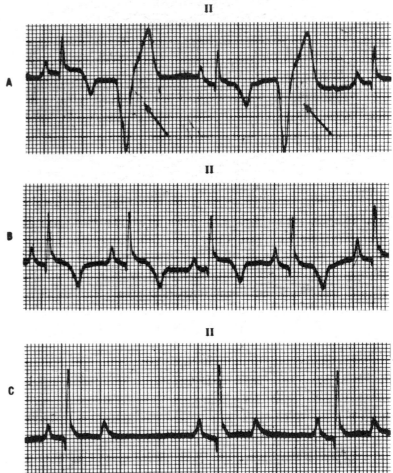

Another area for ECG application is in patients having seizures — usually to help rule in or rule out the role of cardiac disease in the production of the seizure. Bradydysrhythmias (slow heart rates) and tachydysrhythmias (fast heart rates) have both been associated with seizures or syncope (fainting), or both. Electrocardiography is also an important part of determining the therapeutic plan for cancer patients, particularly when cardiotoxic drugs (such as doxorubicin) are being considered for chemotherapy. If the patient is already receiving such drugs, ECG monitoring prior to each treatment is strongly recommended, as the toxic effects are often cumulative.

In summary, the ECG is a valuable tool in many aspects of patient care and in a variety of circumstances. The veterinarian–veterinary technician patient care team should recognize the benefits and limitations of electrocardiography and use them as completely as possible.

Key Words Review

Dilation Enlargement of the chamber size of the heart.

Hypertrophy Thickening of the heart muscle.

Dysrhythmia Any abnormal heartbeat sequence.

Pulse Deficit Failure to detect an arterial pulse immediately following each heart beat.

Proarrhythmic Effect Ability of a drug to cause worsening of a dysrhythmia when it is being administered to correct the dysrhythmia.

Traumatic Myocarditis Injury to the heart muscle as a result of trauma to the body.

Bradydysrhythmia Abnormal, slow heart rate.

Tachydysrhythmia Abnormal, rapid heart rate.

Syncope A fainting spell, usually beginning and ending in a matter of seconds.

Seizure Loss of consciousness and control, resulting in uncontrolled muscular movements often accompanied by urination, defecation, and salivation.

Cardiotoxic Drug Any drug that causes damage to the myocardium or specialized conducting tissues of the heart.

Metabolic Disease Any disease condition that results in derangement of the body's electrolyte or acid-base status.

References

Bolton, GR: Prevention and treatment of cardiovascular emergencies during anesthesia and surgery. Vet Clin North Am (Small Animal Practice) 25:411, 1972.

Edwards, NJ: Bolton's Handbook of Canine and Feline Electrocardiography, ed 2. Philadelphia, WB Saunders, 1987.

Tilley, LP: Essentials of Canine and Feline Electrocardiography, ed 2. Philadelphia, Lea and Febiger, 1985.

CHAPTER

5

Recognition and Elimination of Artifacts

Every veterinary technician needs to be capable of obtaining an artifact-free ECG tracing as the first step toward accurate assessment of the patient's cardiac electrophysiologic state. Because artifacts mimic or obscure the normal waveforms, it is critical that each tracing be as free of artifacts as possible. The most common artifacts in veterinary electrocardiography are respiratory, patient movement, and electrical artifacts. Less commonly encountered artifacts include weak signals, no waveforms, intermittent loss of signal, poorly defined baseline, and inadequate frequency response of the unit.

RESPIRATORY ARTIFACTS

When animals breathe, even normally, there is some body movement that results in both the forelegs and rear legs and their attached electrodes to move up and down during inspiration and expiration. This is particularly true when patients are restrained in the recumbent right lateral position. Obviously deep respirations, panting, or dyspnea will exaggerate this movement causing marked fluctuations of the baseline that obscure or alter the appearance of the P-QRS-T complex (Fig. 5–1). Respiratory artifacts can be minimized by calming the patient, placing a hand over the thorax to minimize excursions, or closing the patient's mouth, forcing it to breathe through its nasal passages. Towels, cotton rolls, or paper towel rolls may be placed between the legs and the

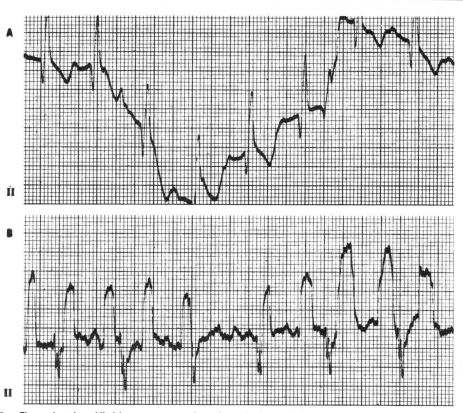

Figure 5 – 1 ▪ These two lead II strips are examples of respiratory artifacts. *A*, Each time this dog took a breath, the tracing would shift downward, making it impossible to keep the complexes on the paper. *B*, This dog was panting, which caused the baseline to jump with each breath. This gives the false impression of abnormal beats. (Paper speed = 50 mm/sec, 1 cm = 1 mv.) (From Edwards, NJ: Bolton's Handbook of Canine and Feline Electrocardiography, ed 2. Philadelphia, WB Saunders, 1987, with permission.)

electrodes to minimize leg movement. The patient's cable can also be secured to the table in such a way as to minimize movement of the cable or electrodes or both. If the patient is having respiratory embarrassment, and particularly if breathing movements become exaggerated when the patient is placed in right lateral recumbency, record the ECG in whatever position the patient is most comfortable. Patient position will not affect the analysis of heart rate or rhythm. If measurements and axis determinations are important, the ECG can be repeated at a later date in the standard position.

PATIENT MOVEMENT ARTIFACTS

Muscular tremors, twitches, or gross body movement will produce varied deviations in the baseline. Fine muscular tremors usually produce small irregular movements throughout the baseline that resemble P waves (Fig. 5–2). Major patient movement, such as struggling or the foot stomping or tail swishing of a horse during fly season, usually results in an abrupt movement of the stylus of such a magnitude that it may actually move off the paper (Fig. 5–3).

A purring artifact may be seen in cats, which is usually a short period of small irregular movements in the baseline interspaced with periods of minimal baseline deviation. If in doubt, these are easily correlated with the purring sound and can be identified on the ECG tracing by pressing the marker button during the period of purring (Fig. 5–4).

Patient movement artifacts can be minimized by making sure the patient is in as comfortable a position as possible. Padding the table with a piece of four-inch foam protected by a vinyl cover may be helpful in small patients.

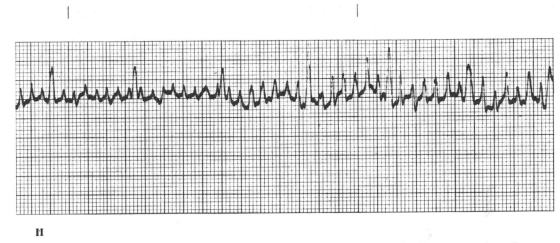

II

Figure 5–2 ▪ This lead II ECG was recorded from a 5-year-old standard poodle. The uneven baseline resembling many P waves between QRS complexes is being caused by muscular tremor. (Paper speed = 50 mm/sec; 1 cm = 1 mv.) (From Edwards, NJ: Bolton's Handbook of Canine and Feline Electrocardiography, ed 2. Philadelphia, WB Saunders, 1987, with permission.)

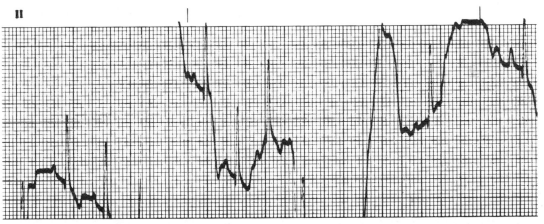

II

Figure 5–3 ▪ This lead II ECG tracing is being taken on a German shepherd. Notice what happened to the baseline when quick sudden patient movement occurred.

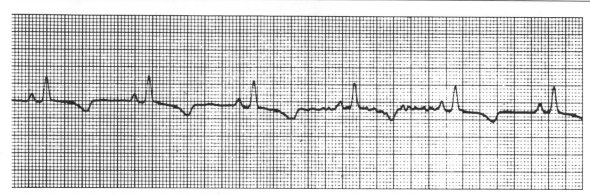

Figure 5–4 ▪ This lead II ECG tracing was recorded from a 1-year-old Siamese cat being evaluated for a heart murmur. Note the sudden change in baseline beginning with the fourth P-QRS-T complex from the left. This is purring artifact. (From Edwards, NJ: Bolton's Handbook of Canine and Feline Electrocardiography, ed 2. Philadelphia, WB Saunders, 1987, with permission.)

Application of wipe-on fly sprays or wrapping the tail may help alleviate muscular twitching in larger animals. Because nervousness is another important reason for patient movement, taking the time to calm the patient and gain its confidence before attaching the electrodes is beneficial, regardless of the species. Occasionally readjustment of the electrodes may help relieve discomfort and hence minimize patient movement. Direct pressure on the body of small animal patients may also help alleviate patient movement. If all else fails, reduction of the amplitude to half sensitivity (0.5 cm = 1 mv) will reduce the amplitude of the artifacts; remember, however, that it will reduce the amplitude of the P-QRS-T complex as well. When attaching electrode clips to the horse or cow, pinching the site immediately before attaching the clip helps to alleviate discomfort and subsequent patient movement.

ELECTRICAL ARTIFACTS

The most common electrical artifact is that caused by 60-cycle electrical interference. The 60-cycle artifact looks like a uniform saw-toothed, up-and-down movement of the baseline throughout the ECG tracing. If one were to count these up-and-down movements, there would be 60 waves per second uniformly throughout the tracing. However, they are difficult to count and that is not necessary in order to recognize this artifact (Fig. 5–5). Sixty-cycle artifacts make an ECG tracing all but unreadable unless the 60-cycle waveform is very small. Consequently it should be considered mandatory to eliminate this artifact from any ECG. The following checklist may be helpful in eliminating electrical interference. The items are listed in order of importance.

1. Make sure that the clips are clean and attached tightly to the cables. Rust and corrosion that build up on the clips can be removed with sandpaper. The clips should be replaced occasionally, depending on their use and condition.

2. Check the leads as they are attached to the patient. Try to attach them firmly, with good skin contact. The leads should be wetted adequately but not excessively with alcohol. If the leads are wetted too vigorously, the hair may become so wet that electrical contact is established between the two clips or between the clips and table. This problem can be corrected by wadding dry paper towels between the legs to insulate the clips from one another. The table beneath the animal should also be kept as dry as possible to avoid conductivity problems.

3. Make sure that the clips do not touch each other. Paper towels wadded between the legs are also helpful in this respect.

4. Make sure that the holder is not touching any of the clips. The body is an excellent conductive medium.

5. Check the ground cord and attach it to various ground contacts.

II

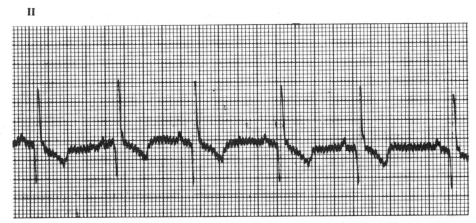

Figure 5-5 ▪ When this lead II ECG was recorded, the dog was not properly grounded, and the regular saw-toothed artifact of 60-cycle electrical interference is seen. Such an error makes measurements and observations difficult. Here it is hard to measure the P wave or to see if an S wave is present. (Paper speed = 50 mm/sec, 1 cm = 1 mv.) (From Edwards, NJ: Bolton's Handbook of Canine and Feline Electrocardiography, ed 2. Philadelphia, WB Saunders, 1987, with permission.)

the equipment manual or the customer service representative of the company manufacturing your ECG machine.

Weak signals, no waveforms, intermittent loss of signals, poorly defined baselines and inadequate frequency responses are usually the results of defects in the patient's cable, the stylus, or the ECG unit itself. If any of these occurs, first check the electrode–patient cable contact and the patient cable–ECG unit contact. If no abnormality can be found, increase the stylus heat and/or clean any dirt or accumulated material from the ECG paper from the stylus. Be sure to have the machine turned off and allow the stylus to cool before touching it, if running the paper drive with increased stylus heat fails to clean the stylus. An extra patient cable is a handy thing to have when trying to diagnose and eliminate these artifacts. Simply replacing the old cable with the spare one will help isolate the problem to the cable or the unit. If the unit is at fault, it should be checked by the manufacturer or an authorized service representative. Do not attempt any repair other than replacement of the stylus at any time for any reason.

6. If the machine has a ground switch, flip it back and forth to see which setting is best for producing a smooth steady tracing. Turning the plug around in the wall socket sometimes helps.

7. Turn out the room light. Fluorescent lights may be especially troublesome.

8. Place the patient or even the entire table on a rubber mat or a wool blanket for insulation.

9. Unplug any electrical appliances that are connected to the same circuit as the electrocardiograph (e.g., x-ray view boxes, centrifuges, radios).

10. Change animal holders. Occasionally, on certain days, some people conduct electricity, and a change of holders may eliminate the 60-cycle interference.

11. Remove any electrical watches from the vicinity. It is best not to wear a watch, because the electrocardiograph has a powerful electromagnetic field that could cause a watch to malfunction.

12. If all else fails, move to a different room and review the entire checklist.

13. Move the electrocardiograph to another building.

14. If 60-cycle interference persists, consult

SELF-ASSESSMENT

Evaluate the following ECG tracings and determine what artifacts are present and how you would correct them. The answers are located in the Appendix.

Case 5 – 1 *(Fig. 5 – 6):*

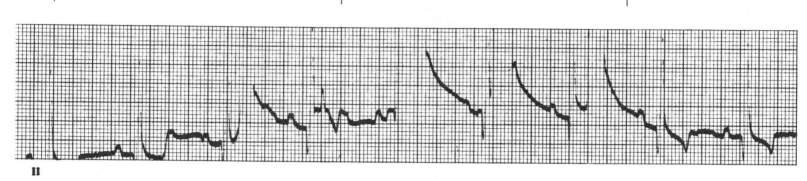

Figure 5 – 6 ▪ This lead II ECG tracing was recorded from a male standard poodle. (1 cm = 1 mv; paper speed 50 = mm/sec.) (From Edwards, NJ: Bolton's Handbook of Canine and Feline Electrocardiography, ed 2. Philadelphia, WB Saunders, 1987, with permission.)

Questions

1. Is this ECG tracing acceptable?
2. What artifacts, if any, are present?
3. What could you do to improve this situation?

Case 5–2 *(Fig. 5–7 A, B):*

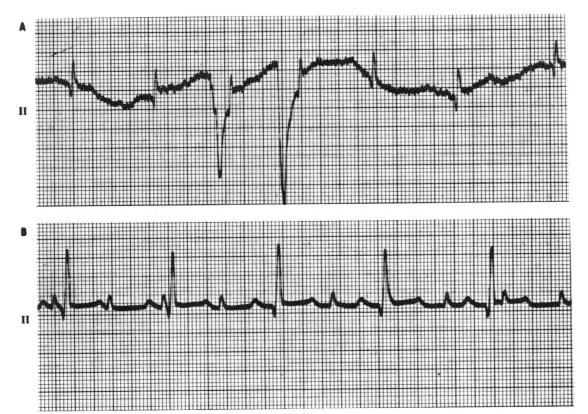

Questions

1. How many artifacts can you identify in the lead II ECG tracing in Figure 5–7A, recorded from a dog?
2. Are any artifacts present on the lead II ECG tracing in Figure 5–7B recorded from a dog (not the same patient as in Fig. 5–7A)? If so, what are they?

Figure 5–7 ▪ *A,* This lead II ECG tracing was recorded from a mixed breed dog with a history of syncope (fainting). (1 cm = 1 mv; paper speed = 50 mm/sec.) (From Edwards, NJ: Bolton's Handbook of Canine and Feline Electrocardiography, ed 2. Philadelphia, WB Saunders, 1987, with permission.)
B, This lead II ECG tracing was recorded from a mixed breed dog with a history of sudden onset of abdominal swelling (ascites). (1 cm = 1 mv; paper speed = 50 mm/sec.) (From Edwards, NJ: Bolton's Handbook of Canine and Feline Electrocardiography, ed 2. Philadelphia, WB Saunders, 1987, with permission.)

Case 5–3 *(Fig. 5–8):*

1. What artifact is present?
2. How would you correct it?

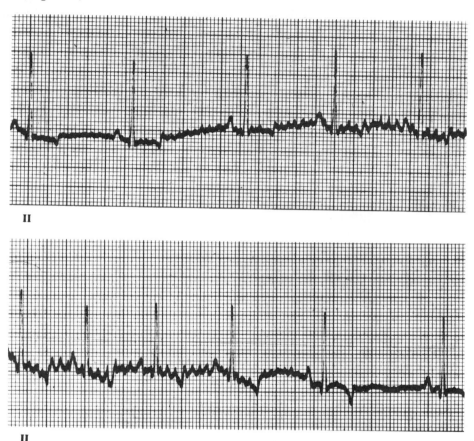

II

II

Figure 5–8 ▪ These two lead II ECG continuous tracings were recorded from a miniature poodle with a loud heart murmur. (1 cm = 1 mv, paper speed = 50 mm/sec.) (From Edwards, NJ: Bolton's Handbook of Canine and Feline Electrocardiography, ed 2. Philadelphia, WB Saunders, 1987, with permission.)

Case 5-4 *(Fig. 5-9, A, B)*

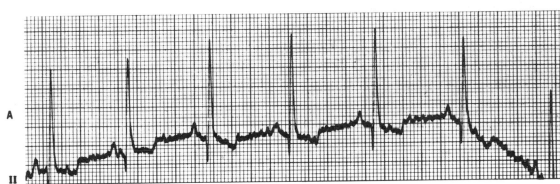

A

II

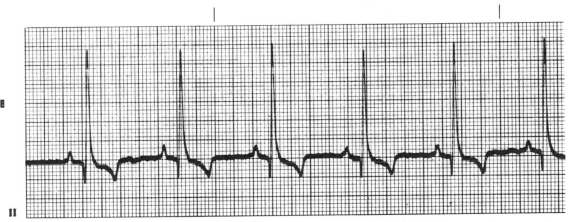

B

II

Figure 5-9 ▪ *A, B*, These two lead II ECG tracings were recorded from an Irish terrier dog with an enlarged heart seen on thoracic radiography. (From Edwards, NJ: Bolton's Handbook of Canine and Feline Electrocardiography, ed 2. Philadelphia, WB Saunders, 1987, with permission.)

Question

1. What artifacts are present in this lead II ECG recorded from an Irish terrier (top strip)?

Case 5 – 5 *(Fig. 5 – 10 A, B):*

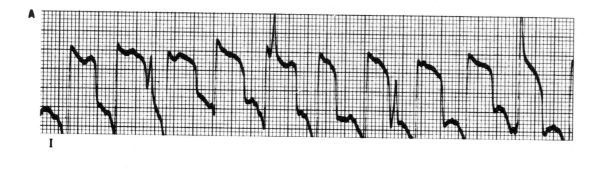

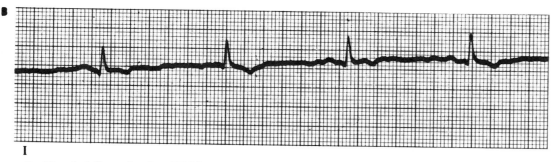

Figure 5 – 10 ▪ *A, B,* These two lead I ECG tracings were recorded from an aged English pointer dog with a history of failing to hunt well. (1 cm = 1 mv; paper speed = 50 mm/sec.) (From Edwards, NJ: Bolton's Handbook of Canine and Feline Electrocardiography, ed 2. Philadelphia, WB Saunders, 1987, with permission.)

Questions

1. What artifact is present in the top tracing?
2. Can you list some techniques that might have been used to record the lower tracing?

Case 5 – 6 *(Fig. 5 – 11):*

Questions
1. What artifact is present?
2. What steps would you take to correct the problem?

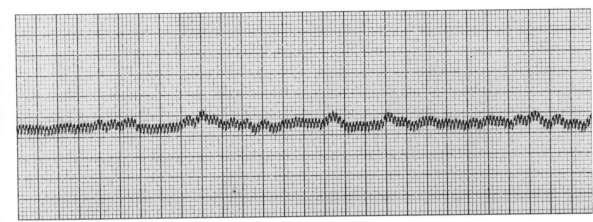

Figure 5 – 11 ▪ This lead II ECG tracing was being recorded from a 24-year-old stable horse gelding with a history of not wanting to complete trial rides. (1 cm = 1 mv; paper speed = 50 mm/sec.)

Key Words Review

Artifact Any movement of the ECG stylus not caused by the electrical output of the heart.

Respiratory Artifact Movement in the ECG baseline associated with breathing.

Patient Movement Artifact Gross movement in the ECG baseline caused by patient movement.

Muscular Tremor Artifact Fine up-and-down movement in the ECG baseline caused by muscular tremors, resulting in a jagged baseline.

60-Cycle Artifact Uniform sine wave alterations of the baseline caused by electrical interference.

Purring Artifact Intermittent saw-toothed irregularity in the ECG baseline associated with purring in the cat.

References

Blowers, MG, and Sims, RS: How to Read an ECG, ed 4. Oradell, NJ, Medical Economics, 1988.

Conover, MB: Pocket Guide to Electrocardiography, ed 2. St Louis, CV Mosby, 1990.

Edwards, NJ: Bolton's Handbook of Canine and Feline Electrocardiography, ed 2. Philadelphia, WB Saunders, 1987.

Kelly, WJ: ECG Interpretation. Senior Editor, Clinical Skillbuilders. Springhouse, PA, Springhouse Corp, 1990.

CHAPTER

6

Electrocardiographic Measurements

Each heartbeat is preceded by an electrical stimulus that initiates the mechanical contraction of the cardiac musculature. The electrocardiogram (ECG) records that electrical stimulus and as such is made up of five major waves — P, Q, R, S, and T — and the periods of time between waves — P-R interval, P-R segment, S-T segment, and Q-T interval (Fig. 6–1). These waves, intervals, and segments are measured to provide diagnostic information about the size and health of the heart and encompass the science of electrocardiography.

There are five basic steps in the process of interpreting an ECG: determining the heart rate, determining the heart rhythm, determining the mean electrical axis, measuring the amplitude and duration of the waveforms, segments and intervals, and applying miscellaneous criteria (Table 6–1). The measurement of amplitude and duration of the waveforms, segments, and intervals is broken down into six steps:

1. Measurement of the P wave
2. Measurement of the P-R interval
3. Measurement of the QRS complex
4. Measurement of the S-T segment
5. Measurement of the T wave
6. Measurement of the Q-T interval.

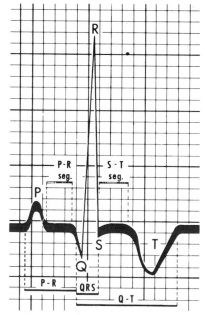

Figure 6–1 ▪ A schematic representation is shown of the different ECG waveforms, intervals, and segments that demonstrate the electrical energy associated with mechanical contraction and relaxation of the heart muscle. ((From Edwards, NJ: Bolton's Handbook of Canine and Feline Electrocardiography, ed 2. Philadelphia, WB Saunders, 1987, with permission.)

TABLE 6–1 ▪ Five Basic Steps of ECG Assessment

1. Determine heart rate
   a. "10 or 20 method"
   b. "1500 or 3000 method"
   c. "Sequence method"
2. Determine heart rhythm
   a. "Paper-and-pencil method"
   b. "Caliper melthod"
3. Determine the mean electrical axis
   a. "Any two lead method"
   b. "Quadrant method"
   c. "Isoelectric lead method"
4. Measurement of waveforms, intervals, and segments
   a. Amplitude
   b. Duration
5. Application of miscellaneous criteria
   a. Criteria for enlargement
   b. Conduction abnormalities

DETERMINING HEART RATE

The lead II rhythm strip is usually the best location for determining the heart rate. Three methods are routinely used. The first, called the "10 or 20 method," uses a series of hash marks at the top or bottom of the paper (Fig. 6–2). These marks are spaced so that at 50 mm/sec paper speed they are 1½ sec apart (3 sec apart when using a paper speed of 25 mm/sec). To estimate the heart rate per minute, count the number of complexes that occur in 3 sec and multiply by 20 or the number of complexes that occur in 6 sec and multiply by 10, depending on the ECG paper speed (25 mm/sec; multiply by 10; 50 mm/sec, multiply by 20). In Figure 6–3 it can be seen that there are four P-QRS-T complexes that occur over a 3-sec time span. Hence the heart rate/minute would be 4 × 20 = 80. It is sometimes helpful to count the P-wave rate and the QRS rate individually if a dysrhythmia is present.

The second method of determining heart rate/minute is called the "1500 or 3000 method." It is particularly useful if the rate is very regular. With this method, the number of small boxes from R wave to R wave are

Figure 6–2 ▪ Along the top of this ECG recording paper are marks seen at regular intervals throughout (three of them are shown here). When the paper is run at 50 mm/sec, the time between two marks is 1½ seconds. To estimate the heart rate, count the number of complexes in 3 sec and multiply by 20. When the paper is run at 25 mm/sec, the time between the two marks becomes 3 sec. To estimate the heart rate at this speed, count the number of complexes in 6 sec and multiply by 10. (From Edwards, NJ: Bolton's Handbook of Canine and Feline Electrocardiography, ed 2. Philadelphia, WB Saunders, 1987, with permission.)

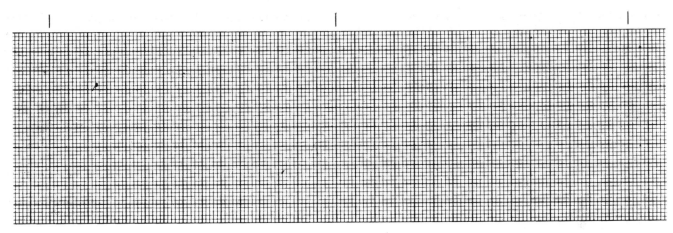

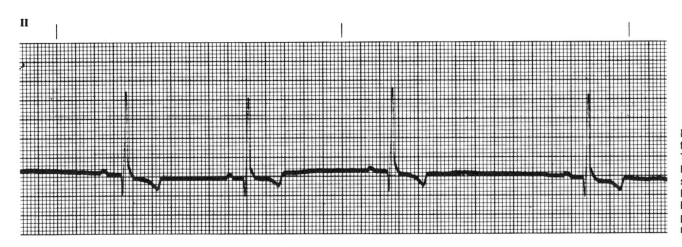

Figure 6–3 ▪ In this tracing, there are four complexes that occur in 3 seconds. Therefore, this dog's heart rate is 80 beats/min. (Paper speed = 50 mm/sec, 1 cm = 1 mv.) (From Edwards, NJ: Bolton's Handbook of Canine and Feline Electrocardiography, ed 2. Philadelphia, WB Saunders, 1987, with permission.)

II

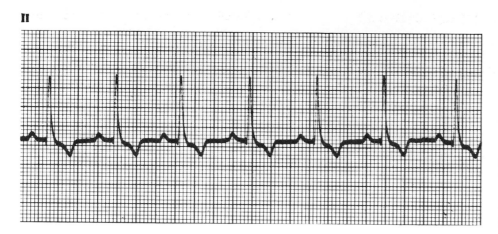

Figure 6–4 ▪ In this ECG tracing, the heart rate can be determined by counting the number of small boxes in each R-R interval and dividing into 3000. The R-R interval ranges from 16 to 18 small boxes, so the heart rate is 166 to 187 beats/min. (Paper speed = 50 mm/sec, 1 cm = 1 mv.) (From Edwards, NJ: Bolton's Handbook of Canine and Feline Electrocardiography, ed 2. Philadelphia, WB Saunders, 1987, with permission.)

Figure 6–5 ▪ This is the same ECG tracing as in Figure 6–4. Using the sequence method, the second R wave from the left peaks very near a heavy black line. If we assign 600, 300, 200, 150, 120, and 100 beats per minute to the succeeding heavy black vertical lines, we see the next R wave falls between the lines representing 200 and 150 beats/min. Consequently, a quick assessment of heart rate would be 175 beats/min. Closer inspection reveals the succeeding P wave (third from the left) falls closer to the 200 beats/min line (between 175 and 200), allowing a more precise estimate of 188 beats/min. (Paper speed = 50 mm/sec, 1 cm = 1 mv.) (From Edwards, NJ: Bolton's Handbook of Canine and Feline Electrocardiography, ed 2. Philadelphia, WB Saunders, 1987, with permission.)

II

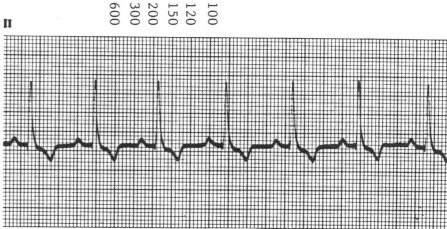

counted. There are 3000 small boxes/minute when the ECG is recorded at 50 mm/sec and 1500 small boxes/minute when the ECG is recorded at 25 mm/sec. Consequently at 50 mm/sec the number of small boxes counted between two R waves is divided into 3000 to calculate the heart rate/minute. At a paper speed of 25 mm/sec the number of boxes between two R waves is divided into 1500. The distance between two R waves is called the R-R interval. The "1500 or 3000 method" is a more accurate way of determining a precise heart rate, but it is more time consuming than the "10 or 20 method" and works best when the R-R interval is nearly uniform. Contrast the R-R intervals of Figure 6–3 with those of Figure 6–4. Compare the wide range of calculated heart rate using the "1500 or 3000 method" for the ECG in Figure 6–3.

The third method of determining heart rate/minute is the "sequence method." First, find an R wave that peaks on a heavy black line. At a paper speed of 50 mm/sec, assign the following numbers to the next six heavy black lines: 600, 300, 200, 150, 120, and 100, respectively. At a paper speed of 25 mm/sec these numbers would become in the same order 300, 150, 100, 75, 60, 50. Find the next R-wave peak and estimate the heart rate/minute based on the number assigned to the nearest heavy black line (Fig. 6–5). The "sequence method" is a rapid method of determining heart rate once you become familiar with it.

DETERMINING HEART RHYTHM

To assess the rhythm, a systematic evaluation of both atrial and ventricular rhythm should be performed. Visual inspection together with either the "paper-and-pencil method" or the "caliper method" should be done. A regular repetitive sequence of a P wave followed by a short pause (P-R segment), then a QRS complex followed by another short pause (S-T segment), and finally a T wave should occur on the normal ECG (Fig. 6–6). This sequence should remain consistent throughout the ECG. Five basic questions should be asked when determining the heart rhythm:

1. Is the heart rate normal or abnormal?
2. Is the rhythm regular or irregular?
3. Can I identify P waves and QRS com-

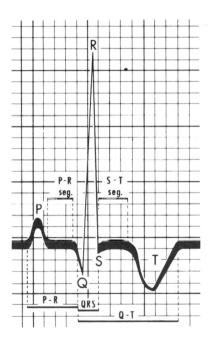

Figure 6–6 ▪ Shown is a schematic representation of the different ECG waveforms, intervals, and segments that demonstrate the electrical energy associated with mechanical contraction and relaxation of the heart muscle. (From Edwards, NJ: Bolton's Handbook of Canine and Feline Electrocardiography, ed 2. Philadelphia, WB Saunders, 1987, with permission.)

plexes? (Is there a P wave before every QRS complex and a QRS complex following every P wave?)

4. Are all P waves consistently related to the QRS complex? (Are the P-R intervals all the same?)

5. Do all the P waves look alike? (Do all the QRS complexes look alike?)

If you answer "no" to any of these questions, some type of dysrhythmia is present. In general, the more "no" answers, the more serious the dysrhythmia and the more significant the need for correction.

TABLE 6–2 ■ Normal Heart Rates (beats per minute)

Dog	
Adult	70–160
Giant breed	60–140
Toy breed	70–180
Puppy	70–220
Cat	90–240
Ferret	180–240
Horse	26–50
Miniature Horse	40–70
Pony	35–40
Cow	30–50
Calf	90–130
Sheep	80–100
Goat	90–130
Llama	40–70

Normal or Abnormal Heart Rate

Once the heart rate is determined, a simple check comparing results with published normal values for each species will allow you to determine the answer (Table 6–2).

Regular or Irregular Rhythm

Visual inspection coupled with either the "pencil-and-paper method" or the "caliper method" may be used to determine regularity or irregularity. Visual inspection may be all that is required (Fig. 6–7). A more precise assessment with either the "pencil-and-paper method" or the "caliper method" may be necessary in other instances (Fig. 6–8). The "paper-and-pencil method" of rhythm assessment is performed as follows (Fig. 6–9): Place the ECG strip on a flat surface. Place the straight edge of a piece of paper along the baseline. Next, move the paper upward until it nears the peak of the R wave, when determining ventricular rhythm, or near the peak of the P wave, when determining atrial rhythm. With a pencil, make dots or hash marks near the edge of the paper where it contacts the peak of the R (or P) wave of the first two or three R (or P) waves. Now, move the paper across the strip from left to right, lining up the first dot or hash mark with succeeding R (or P) waves. If the rhythm is regular (normal sinus rhythm), all of the dots or hash marks will fall on the peak of

each succeeding R (or P) wave. If the rhythm is irregular, the dots or hash marks will miss the R (or P) wave peak.

The "caliper method" utilizes the same principle (Fig. 6–10). With the ECG strip on a flat surface, place one point of the caliper on the peak of the first R (or P) wave and adjust the caliper legs so that the other point is on the peak of the next R (or P) wave. This distance is the R-R interval (or P-P interval). Now move the calipers, placing one point on the next (second) R (or P) wave peak and see how close the other leg of the calipers comes to the peak of the third R (or P) wave. Do this across several complexes. If the rhythm is regular, the caliper legs will fall precisely on the peaks of successive R (or P) waves. If the rhythm is irregular, the caliper leg will miss landing at the peak of the R wave (or P wave, in the case of measurement of atrial rhythm).

The normal rhythm is sinus in origin (meaning that normal P waves are present and consistently related to every QRS complex). If there is a sinus rhythm that is perfectly regular, it is called a normal sinus rhythm (NSR). If there is a sinus rhythm that is somewhat irregular, it is called sinus arrhythmia (SA). Most normal cats and ferrets have NSR. Normal dogs may have either NSR or SA. Normal horses and cattle often have SA at rest that becomes NSR during or after exercise. Mild variations in P-wave morphology are often associated with SA. This is called a wandering

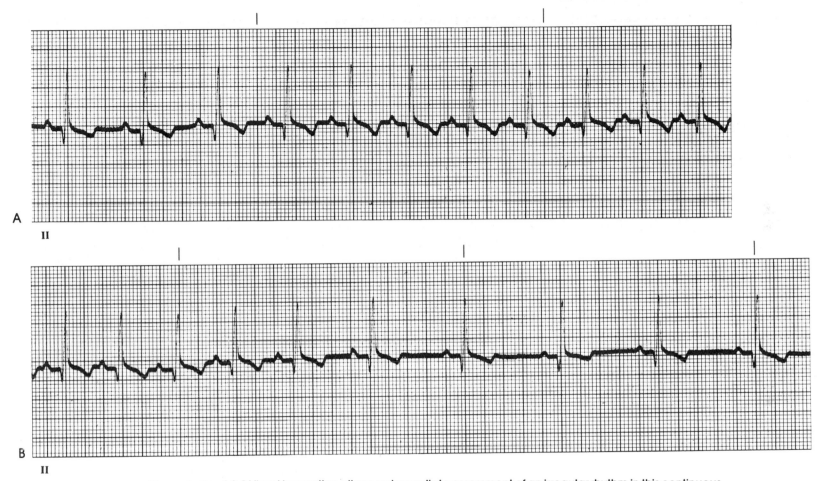

Figure 6–7 ▪ *A* & *B* Visual inspection allows an immediate assessment of an irregular rhythm in this continuous lead II ECG from an old dog with a prostatic abscess. Note how the rhythm changes to a faster rate at the end of the top strip, continues on the beginning of the bottom strip, and then slows toward the end of the bottom strip. Careful observation shows that the P waves during the more rapid heart rate look slightly different than those during slower heart rate. (Paper speed = 50 mm/sec, 1 cm = 1 mv.) (From Edwards, NJ: Bolton's Handbook of Canine and Feline Electrocardiography, ed 2. Philadelphia, WB Saunders, 1987, with permission.)

II

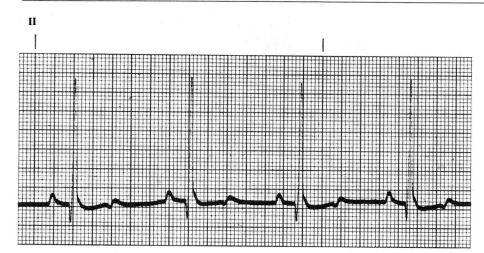

Figure 6–8 ▪ This lead II ECG was recorded from an Old English sheepdog. Note that by using either the pencil-and-paper method or the caliper method there is a slight variation in R-R intervals and P-P intervals on this tracing. This is mild sinus arrhythmia, which is considered normal for this dog. (From Edwards, NJ: Bolton's Handbook of Canine and Feline Electrocardiography, ed 2. Philadelphia, WB Saunders, 1987, with permission.)

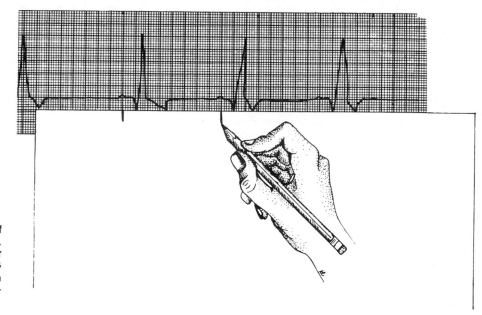

Figure 6–9 ▪ Paper-and-pencil method of rhythm assessment. A piece of paper is placed on the ECG tracing so that its edge is along the baseline. With a pen or pencil, make a dot or hash mark at the peak of the first two or three P waves. Then slide the paper along the remaining portion of the ECG tracing and see whether succeeding P wave peaks line up with the marks on the edge of the paper. R wave regularity can also be checked in this manner, marking the peak of the R wave instead of the P wave.

pacemaker and is considered normal in the presence of SA.

DETERMINING MEAN ELECTRICAL AXIS

A lead axis is an imaginary line drawn between two electrodes. When the main current flow is parallel to the axis of a lead, the resulting QRS complex is the most positive or negative deflection of any of the leads, depending on which direction the current is flowing (Fig. 6–11). Current flowing toward the positive pole of a lead produces a positive complex. Current flowing toward the negative pole of a lead pro-

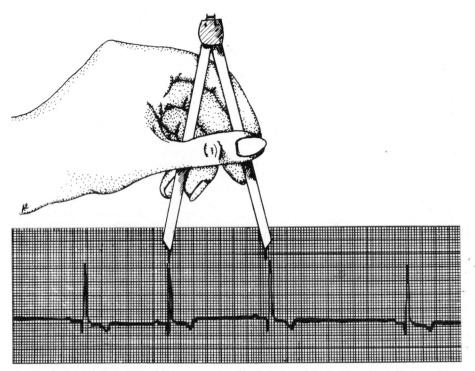

Figure 6–10 ▪ Caliper method of rhythm assessment. Place the points of a set of calipers on the peak of two successive P or R waves. Lock the calipers, and then move them, placing the points on successive P or R waves, depending on which interval (P-P or R-R) is being measured.

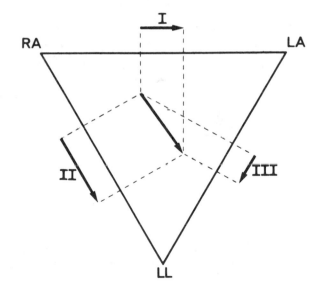

Figure 6–11 ▪ It is apparent that, when the cardiac vector is projected within a triangle representing the three standard limb leads, the longest vector will be projected on the lead most nearly parallel to the cardiac vector (lead II in this case). Similarly, the shortest vector will be projected on the lead most nearly perpendicular to the cardiac vector (lead III). (From Ettinger, SJ, and Suter, PF: Canine Cardiology. WB Saunders, Philadelphia, 1970.)

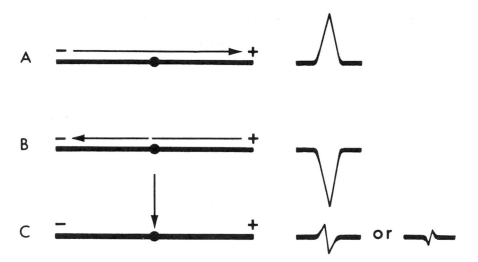

Figure 6–12 ▪ Each lead has a positive pole and a negative pole. *A*, If the vector (or *impulse*) runs toward the positive pole, a positive (upward) deflection occurs; *B*, if the impulse runs toward the negative pole, a negative (downward) deflection results; *C*, if the main impulse runs perpendicular to a lead, that lead records an isoelectric deflection, which may be either a very small recording, or a recording showing an equal amount of positive and negative deflection. Later, when axis is discussed, it will be important to be able to find which lead is isoelectric, because the main vector will be running perpendicular to the isoelectric lead. (From Edwards, NJ: Bolton's Handbook of Canine and Feline Electrocardiography, ed 2. Philadelphia, WB Saunders, 1987, with permission.)

duces a negative complex (Fig. 6–12). When the main current flow is perpendicular to the axis of a lead, an equiphasic (isoelectric) QRS complex is formed. If a number of vectors are combined where the main current flow (mean vector) ranges from parallel to perpendicular depending on the lead being sampled, various-shaped QRS complexes will result. A mean vector on the positive side of the perpendicular yet not parallel with the lead axis produces a complex that is mostly positive, whereas a mean vector on the negative side of the perpendicular yet not parallel with the lead axis produces a complex that is mostly negative (Fig. 6–13). When all six leads of the frontal axis system (I, II, III, aVR, aVL, and aVF) (Bailey six-axis reference system) are used, the mean

vector of all the leads can be determined by assessing the QRS complex of two or more of the leads. This system can be superimposed in the frontal plane to represent the direction of the mean electrical vector generated by the heart. The direction of that vector is termed the "mean electrical axis" (Fig. 6–14). There are three common methods of determining the mean electrical axis:

1. The "any two lead method"
2. The "quadrant method"
3. The "isoelectric lead method."

The "any two lead method" involves selecting any two leads and adding up the total number of positive and negative deflections of one QRS complex in each of the two leads chosen.

The summed value is plotted on each lead and a perpendicular line drawn from each lead at the value point. A line drawn from the center of the axis chart to the point at which the two perpendicular lines meet will indicate the direction of the mean electrical axis. It is then given a plus or minus degree value, based on its position in the Bailey hexagonal reference system (Fig. 6–15).

The "quadrant method" is a rapid method for approximating the mean electrical axis. This method employs the axis of leads I and aVF to divide the frontal plane into four quadrants: 1, +0 – +90; 2, +90 – +180: 3, −180 – −90; 4, −90 – −0 (Fig. 6–16). If the lead I QRS complex is positive (above the baseline), the axis is somewhere in the positive quadrant of lead I. If the QRS complex in aVF is also positive, the axis is somewhere in the positive quadrant of lead aVF. The quadrant in which the two overlap is the quadrant that contains the mean electrical axis. In the example, this is quadrant 1, representing a mean electrical axis somewhere between +0° and +90° (Fig. 6–17).

The "isoelectric lead method" combines ease with accuracy and is probably the most frequently used method for determining the mean electrical axis. The steps are as follows:

1. Find the isoelectric lead or the lead closest to being isoelectric.
2. Use the Bailey six-axis reference system.
3. Determine whether the QRS of the perpendicular lead is positive or negative.
4. Determine the degree value on the positive or negative pole of the perpendicular lead.

Finding an Isoelectric Lead

An isoelectric lead is one in which all the positive and negative deflections of the QRS complex add up to zero. For example, examine Figure 6–18. Leads I, II, III, and aVF are all more positive than negative. Lead aVR is more negative than positive. Lead aVL has an initial small positive deflection of one small box (+1 mv) followed by a negative deflection of approximately four small boxes (−4 mv) and then a positive deflection of approximately three small boxes (+3 mv). Added together (+1, −4, +3), these equal zero, which makes lead aVL the isoelectric lead in this ECG tracing.

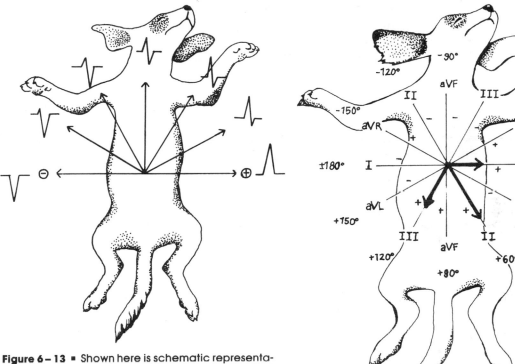

Figure 6–13 ▪ Shown here is schematic representation of changes in shape of the QRS complex that occur when the mean cardiac vector is in various directions compared with the direction of a lead axis (in this case, lead I).

Figure 6–14 ▪ Bailey six-axis reference system superimposed on the dog. Bailey system (leads I, II, III, aVR, aVL, and aVF) for the frontal plane has the lead axes marked in 30° increments from 0° to +180° on the bottom half of the circle and 0° to −180° on the top half of the circle. Note that each lead has a positive and negative pole. This system is seen superimposed on the chest (frontal plane) as the different lead positions "see" the mean vector of electrical activity generated by the heart. In this case, the major current flow is along the lead II axis and is traveling toward the positive pole of lead II. Therefore, the mean electrical axis (major vector or net vector force) in the frontal plane is calculated as +60°.

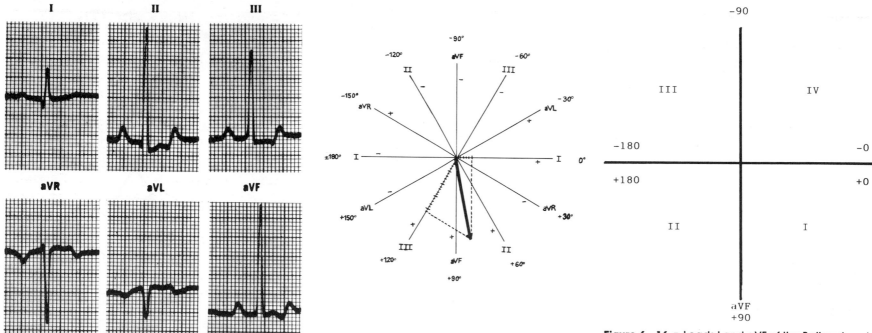

Figure 6–15 ▪ A two-lead method of determining mean electrical axis. Choosing any two limb leads, the positive and negative deflections for one QRS complex in each lead are added and the result plotted along the corresponding axis. Perpendicular lines are then drawn from the value points along each lead and extended until they meet. A line drawn from the center of the axis system to the point where the two perpendicular lines intersect represents the direction of the mean electrical axis.

In this case, leads I and III have been chosen. Lead I has an initial wave deflection of 2 small boxes below the baseline (−2), followed by an R wave of 7 small boxes above the baseline (+7). Adding these two numbers (−2, +7) results in a +5 small boxes, which are plotted out along the lead I axis toward the positive pole (because the net voltage for lead I was +5). In the same manner, lead III has no q and no s wave. The R wave is 21 small boxes tall. Therefore, adding these three results (0, +21, +0) equals +21, which is plotted on the lead III axis in the direction of the positive pole. Perpendicular lines drawn from each of these two points (+5 on the lead I axis and +21 on the lead III axis) intersect at a point corresponding with approximately +75 to 80° on the Bailey six-axis reference system. A line drawn from the center to this point represents the direction and magnitude of the mean electrical axis in the frontal plane. (Modified from Edwards, NJ: Bolton's Handbook of Canine and Feline Electrocardiography, ed 2. Philadelphia, WB Saunders, 1987, with permission.)

Figure 6–16 ▪ Leads I and aVF of the Bailey six-axis reference system are superimposed to produce four quadrants in the quadrant method for determining the mean electrical axis in the frontal plane.

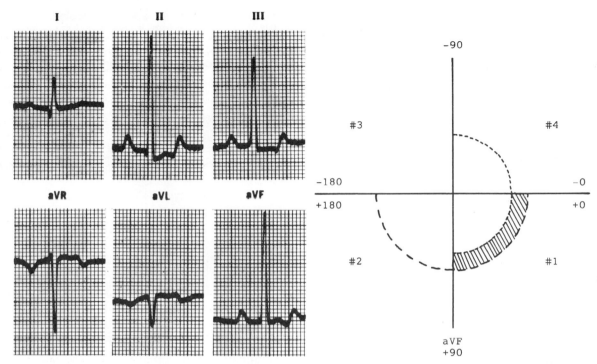

Figure 6–17 ▪ Lead I is positive so the axis is somewhere in the positive half of lead I (*shortest dotted line*). Lead aVF is also positive, so the axis is somewhere in the positive half of lead aVF (*longer dotted line*). The quadrant where they overlap represents the area in which the mean electrical axis is located (+0 to +90 degrees). (Modified from Edwards, NJ: Bolton's Handbook of Canine and Feline Electrocardiography, ed 2. Philadelphia, WB Saunders, 1987, with permission.)

Using the Bailey Six-Axis Reference System

The six-axis reference system superimposes all six frontal leads (review Fig. 6–14). By referring to this diagram, the lead perpendicular to that chosen as being isoelectric can be determined. In Figure 6–18, lead aVL was determined to be isoelectric. Using the Bailey six-axis diagram it can be seen that lead II is that which is perpendicular to lead aVL. Reviewing Figure 6–18, lead II is clearly positive (major deflection above the baseline). By finding the positive pole of lead II on the six-axis reference system, it can be seen it is at +60°. Hence, the mean electrical axis for the ECG depicted in Figure 6–18 is +60°. If lead I is isoelectric, lead aVF would be the perpendicular lead. If lead aVF were positive, the mean electrical axis would be +90° (Fig. 6–24). What would the mean electrical axis be if lead I were isoelectric and lead aVF negative? Referring to Figure 6–14, it can be determined that the mean electrical axis would be −90°.

An additional step is used when no single lead is considered isoelectric. Review Figures 6–19, 6–20, and 6–22. For instance, in Figure 6–22, lead I and lead aVL are the closest to being isoelectric (closest to 0). Lead aVF is perpendicular to lead I and is positive, which would make the mean electrical axis +90°. However, lead I is actually positive (+5), which would shift the mean electrical axis from +90 if lead I was isoelectric (0) toward the positive

In many cases it is not always possible to find a perfectly isoelectric lead. In those cases the lead that is the closest to being isoelectric is chosen (Figs. 6–19, 6–20, 6–21). If two leads are isoelectric or equally close to being isoelectric, then either may be chosen as the isoelectric lead (Fig. 6–22). Occasionally all the leads

will appear isoelectric (Fig. 6–23). In this case, it is not possible to determine the mean electrical axis in the frontal plane (it is most likely in either the transverse or horizontal plane). This is also referred to as an "indeterminate axis" or an "electrically vertical heart."

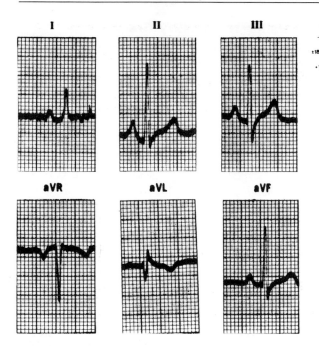

Figure 6–18 ▪ Of the six basic leads in this electrocardiogram, lead aVL is isoelectric. The lead perpendicular to aVL (consult the axis chart, above) is lead II. Lead II on this tracing is positive. This puts the axis at lead II's positive pole, or +60° (see chart). An axis of +60° is normal. (Paper speed = 50 mm/sec, 1 cm = 1 mv.) (From Edwards, NJ: Bolton's Handbook of Canine and Feline Electrocardiography, ed 2. Philadelphia, WB Saunders, 1987, with permission.)

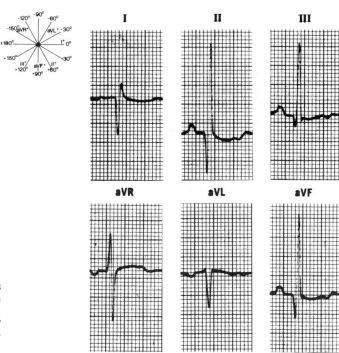

Figure 6–19 ▪ When there is no lead that is perfectly isoelectric, the one most nearly so is used; in this tracing, lead aVR is closest to isoelectric. The perpendicular to lead aVR is lead III (see axis chart). On this tracing, lead III is positive, Lead III's positive pole is at +120°. Because +120° is greater than +100°, this is a right axis deviation, and suggests that the dog has right ventricular hypertrophy. (Paper speed = 50 mm/sec, 1 cm = 1 mv.) (From Edwards, NJ: Bolton's Handbook of Canine and Feline Electrocardiography, ed 2. Philadelphia, WB Saunders, 1987, with permission.)

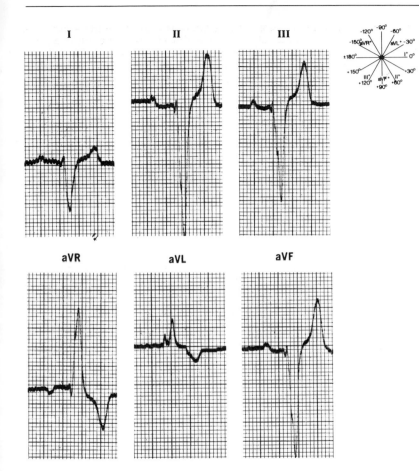

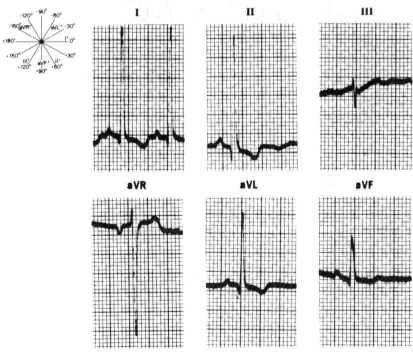

Figure 6–20 ▪ In this electrocardiogram, it is not possible to find a lead that is perfectly isoelectric, so the one most nearly so in this tracing, lead aVL, is used. Lead II is perpendicular to lead aVL and is negative. Lead II's negative pole is at −120° (see chart). This is a severe right ventricular enlargement or right bundle branch block.

Another indication of right ventricular hypertrophy is the presence of an S wave in leads I, II, and III. This is called the S_1, S_2, S_3 pattern, and also indicates right ventricular enlargement. (Paper speed = 50 min/sec, 1 cm = 1 mv.) (From Edwards, NJ: Bolton's Handbook of Canine and Feline Electrocardiography, ed 2. Philadelphia, WB Saunders, 1987, with permission.)

Figure 6–21 ▪ The isoelectric lead in this tracing is lead III. The perpendicular to lead III is lead aVR (see chart). Lead aVR on the tracing is negative, which means that the axis runs toward the negative pole of aVR, or toward +30°. Because +30° is less than +40°, this dog has a left axis deviation, suggesting left ventricular hypertrophy. (Paper speed = 50 min/sec, 1 cm = 1 mv.) (From Edwards, NJ: Bolton's Handbook of Canine and Feline Electrocardiography, ed 2. Philadelphia, WB Saunders, 1987, with permission.)

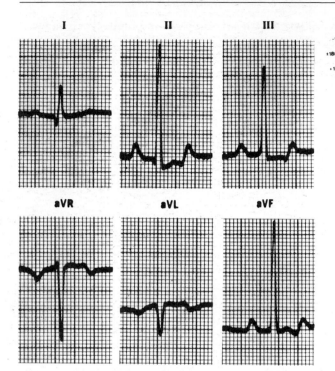

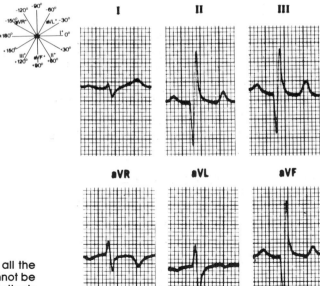

Figure 6–22 ▪ In this tracing, no lead is perfectly isoelectric, but lead I and lead aVL are both equally close. If lead I is used, the perpendicular is aVF and, because aVF is positive the axis would be +90° (normal). If lead aVL is used as isoelectric, lead II is perpendicular and is positive, indicating a +60° axis, which is also normal. If the two are averaged, the result is +75°. Either way, the axis is still normal. (Paper speed = 50 mm/sec, 1 cm = 1 mv.) (From Edwards, NJ: Bolton's Handbook of Canine and Feline Electrocardiography, ed 2. Philadelphia, WB Saunders, 1987, with permission.)

Figure 6–23 ▪ Occasionally a tracing such as this one is recorded in which all the leads are isoelectric. This is termed an electrically vertical heart, and axis cannot be determined. (Paper speed = 50 mm/sec, 1 cm = 1 mv.) (From Edwards, NJ: Bolton's Handbook of Canine and Feline Electrocardiography, ed 2. Philadelphia, WB Saunders, 1987, with permission.)

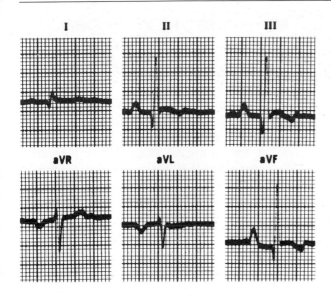

Figure 6–24 ▪ In this electrocardiogram, lead I is isoelectric. On the axis chart, lead aVF is perpendicular to lead I. Because lead aVF is positive on this tracing, the axis runs toward aVF's positive pole, or +90°. An axis of +90° is normal. (Paper speed = 50 min/sec, 1 cm = 1 mv.) (From Edwards, NJ: Bolton's Handbook of Canine and Feline Electrocardiography, ed 2. Philadelphia, WB Saunders, 1987, with permission.)

pole of lead I. A more accurate estimate would be +75° to +80°. On this same ECG tracing, aVL is actually negative (−4). This would shift the axis from +60° (lead II is the perpendicular lead and it is positive) toward the negative pole of aVL (review Figure 6–14) but not past +90° because lead I is positive. The mean electrical axis is approximately +75° to +80° — the same as was determined using lead I as the closest to isoelectric. Close examination of the six-axis reference diagram reveals the positive pole of lead aVL is at −30° and the negative pole is at +150°. Likewise, the positive pole of lead aVR is at −150° and the negative pole is at −30°. These are the only two leads with positive poles having negative values and negative poles having negative values and negative poles hav-

ing positive values. Care must be exercised to avoid confusing the positive pole of these leads with the negative degree value assigned to them.

An approximation of the mean electrical axis in the frontal plane can sometimes be made by finding the lead that is the most positive. The mean electrical axis usually points toward the general direction of the positive pole of the lead. Whichever method is selected for determining the mean electrical axis, the results should be the same.

What is the significance of the mean electrical axis? Normally, the mean electrical axis in the frontal plane for the dog is between +40° and +100°, and for the cat between ±0° and

±180° (Fig. 6–25). If the patient has left ventricular enlargement the mean electrical axis will shift toward the left arm; this is called left axis deviation (Fig. 6–26A). If the axis shifts to the right, past +100° for the dog or past ±180° for the cat, right axis deviation exists and indicates right ventricular enlargement (Fig. 6–26B). If both ventricles are enlarged, the axis often remains within the normal range.

The electrical axis is a reasonably dependable parameter for assessing significant unilateral ventricular enlargement. In the dog, the magnitude of the axis deviation correlates with the severity of the ventricular enlargement. In the cat, however, the mean electrical axis is much less reliable as an indicator of chamber enlargement. It does provide an index of suspicion, though, which may be further evaluated by physical examination, radiography, or echocardiography. Determination of the mean electrical axis in the frontal plane of the horse and cow is not routinely performed because the major vectors are in the transverse and horizontal planes. Reference values for mean electrical axis for the ferret are not currently available.

Conduction defects of the anterior fascicle of the left bundle branch usually shift the axis to a point between −30° and −90°. Conduction defects of the right bundle branch usually shift the axis to a point between −150° and −90°. Complete left bundle branch block usually does not extend the axis beyond normal limits in the frontal plane but does cause marked widening of the QRS (>0.08 sec [dog], > 0.06 sec [cat]).

MEASURING THE WAVEFORMS

The following parts of the P-QRS-T sequence are routinely measured: P wave, P-R interval, QRS complex, S-T segment, T wave, and Q-T interval (see Fig. 6–1). Values are determined for the duration (width) and amplitude (height) of the P wave, QRS complex, and T wave. Values are determined for the duration (length) of the P-R interval, S-T segment, and

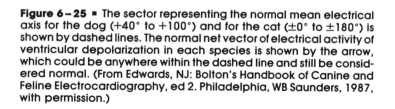

Dog: +40° − 100°

Cat: ±0° − ±180°

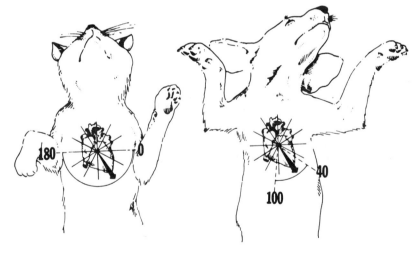

Figure 6–25 ▪ The sector representing the normal mean electrical axis for the dog (+40° to +100°) and for the cat (±0° to ±180°) is shown by dashed lines. The normal net vector of electrical activity of ventricular depolarization in each species is shown by the arrow, which could be anywhere within the dashed line and still be considered normal. (From Edwards, NJ: Bolton's Handbook of Canine and Feline Electrocardiography, ed 2. Philadelphia, WB Saunders, 1987, with permission.)

Q-T interval. *In standard practice all measurements use lead II.* When making the measurements, the waveform duration (width) should be measured from the leading edge of the line at the beginning of the waveform to the leading edge of the line at the conclusion of the waveform, thereby eliminating the tendency to count the width of the line twice which would artifactually increase the measurement. The waveform amplitude (height) should be measured from the top edge of the baseline to the top edge of the waveform. This method too will avoid the counting of the thickness of the line twice and artifactually increasing the amplitude of the waveform. Each of the components of the P-QRS-T sequence will be discussed in detail.

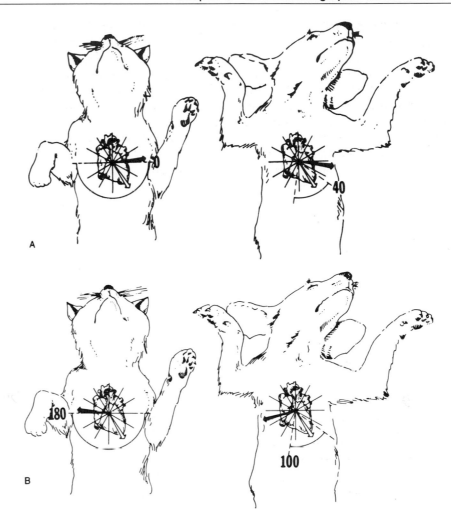

Figure 6–26 ■ *A*, As the left ventricle enlarges, more electrical forces will be generated and their direction will be toward the left. Eventually these new forces become great enough to influence the net vector to shift far enough to the left to be outside the normal sector. When this happens, left axis deviation is said to occur. This is usually a sign of left ventricular enlargement for the dog. In the cat, however, changes in the mean electrical axis are not as reliable. *B*, As the right ventricle enlarges, more electrical forces are generated toward the right, which eventually shifts the net vector beyond the right edge of the normal sector. This is a dependable sign of right ventricular enlargement for the dog, but may not be as specific in the cat. (From Edwards, NJ: Bolton's Handbook of Canine and Feline Electrocardiography, ed 2. Philadelphia, WB Saunders, 1987, with permission.)

The P Wave (Fig. 6–27)

DESCRIPTION

The P wave is the first component of the normal ECG and is produced by depolarization of both right and left atria. P-wave duration (width) represents the time required for atrial conduction and atrial myocardial depolarization. P-wave amplitude (height) represents the amount of current generated during this time.

LOCATION

The P wave precedes the QRS complex and is separated from the QRS complex by the P-R segment.

DURATION

The normal duration (width) of the P wave varies, depending on the species being recorded. There is usually no minimum normal dimension considered because of the varying effects on electrical transmission to the body surface. Instead, the emphasis is on the maximum P-wave duration that is considered normal (Table 6–3). An increase in P-wave duration (width) beyond normal for the species is called *P mitrale* (Figs. 6–28, 6–29, 6–30) and is generally associated with left atrial enlargement in most species.

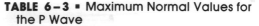

TABLE 6–3 ▪ Maximum Normal Values for the P Wave

	Duration (sec)	Amplitude (mv)
Dog	0.04	0.4
Cat	0.04	0.2
Ferret	0.04	0.1
Horse	0.20	—
Cow	0.10	—

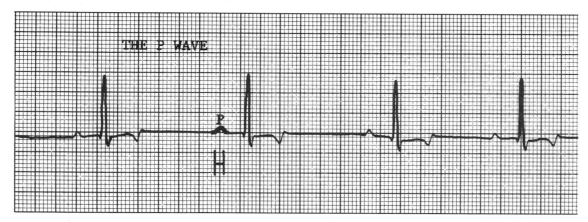

Figure 6–27 ▪ The first component of the normal ECG, the P wave, is produced by atrial depolarization. The P wave has two measurements: duration (width) and amplitude (height). The duration is measured from the leading edge of the stylus mark at the beginning of the P wave as it leaves the baseline to the leading edge of the end of the P wave where it returns to the baseline. The P wave amplitude is measured from the top of the baseline to the peak of the P wave.

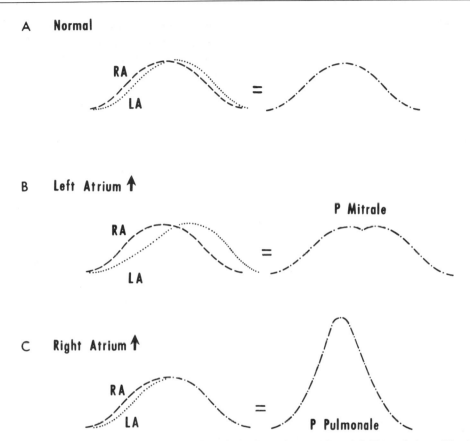

A   **Normal**

RA

LA

=

B   **Left Atrium ↑**

RA

LA

=

P Mitrale

C   **Right Atrium ↑**

RA

LA

=

P Pulmonale

Figure 6–28 ▪ *A,* Normal P wave produced by depolarization of the right and, 0.01 sec later, of the left atria; *B,* when the left atrium enlarges, the impulse takes longer to traverse it, and the left atrial forces are prolonged — this produces a wide P wave (with or without a detectable notch in it) called P mitrale; *C,* when the right atrium enlarges, the impulse takes longer to traverse it, and the right atrial forces are prolonged — this causes a summation of the right and left atrial forces, because they now occur more nearly simultaneously, and a greater millivoltage (taller P wave) is produced. This tall peaked P wave is called P pulmonale. (From Edwards, NJ: Bolton's Handbook of Canine and Feline Electrocardiography, ed 2. Philadelphia, WB Saunders, 1987, with permission.)

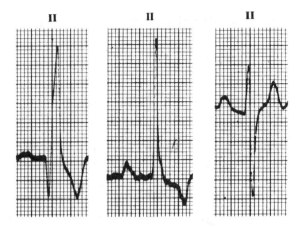

Figure 6–29 ▪ Shown are three examples of P mitrale recorded from three different dogs, indicating left atrial enlargement. In each of the three tracings, the P wave is wider than 0.04 sec (2 boxes). When the P wave becomes wide, it usually has a notch in it, as in these three examples. A notched P wave is not significant unless it is also too wide. (Paper speed = 50 min/sec, 1 cm = 1 mv.) (From Edwards, NJ: Bolton's Handbook of Canine and Feline Electrocardiography, ed 2. Philadelphia, WB Saunders, 1987, with permission.)

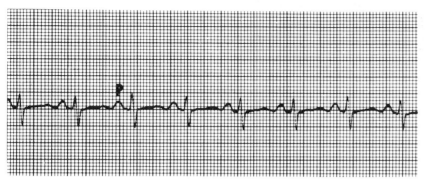

Figure 6-30 ▪ P mitrale in the cat. Note the wide P waves, almost 3 boxes (0.06 sec) wide. The ECG was recorded from a 3-year-old male domestic shorthair (DSH) cat with radiographic evidence of cardiomyopathy. A pronounced left atrial bulge was observed in the ventrodorsal view. (Paper speed = 50 mm/sec, 1 cm = 1 mv.) (From Edwards, NJ: Bolton's Handbook of Canine and Feline Electrocardiography, ed 2. Philadelphia, WB Saunders, 1987, with permission.)

AMPLITUDE

The normal amplitude (height) of the P wave also varies depending on the species being recorded. There are no minimum restrictions placed on the P-wave height in order to be normal; only maximum restrictions exist (Table 6-3). An increase in P-wave amplitude (height) above what is considered normal for the species is called P pulmonale (Figs. 6-28, 6-31, 6-32) and is generally associated with right atrial enlargement in most species.

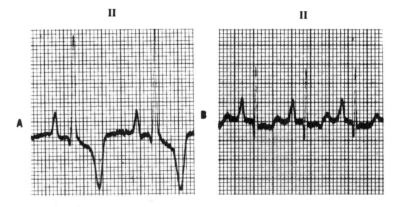

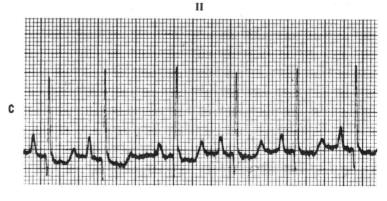

Figure 6-31 ▪ Three different examples of P pulmonale, indicating right atrial enlargement. In each of the three tracings the P waves are consistently taller than 0.4 mv (4 boxes). When they become tall they tend to become peaked. In C the variation in P wave height is called "wandering pacemaker," but the average height of the P waves is 4.3 mv. If the average height of the P waves had been less than 0.4 mv in C, with only an occasional one being too tall, it would not be called P pulmonale. (Paper speed = 50 mm/sec, 1 cm = 1 mv.) (From Edwards, NJ: Bolton's Handbook of Canine and Feline Electrocardiography, ed 2. Philadelphia, WB Saunders, 1987, with permission.)

CONFIGURATION

The normal P wave has a rounded, slightly domed shape. As the heart rate rises, the normal P wave may develop a more peaked shape at the top. In right atrial enlargement, the P waves may also become peaked in appearance (Fig. 6–31). In the horse, cow, and some large breeds of dogs, the normal P wave may also have a slight notch (Fig. 6–33). In left atrial enlargement, P waves often become wide and notched at the top or may have slight irregularities from their normally smooth contour (Figs. 6–29, 6–34).

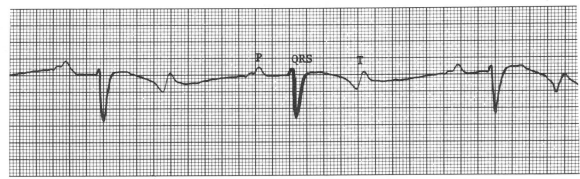

Figure 6–33 ▪ ECG of a horse. This base-apex lead was recorded from a 22-year-old gelding who was a riding stable horse. Note the notching of the P wave; this is normal for the horse. (Paper speed = 50 mm/sec, 1 cm = 1 mv.)

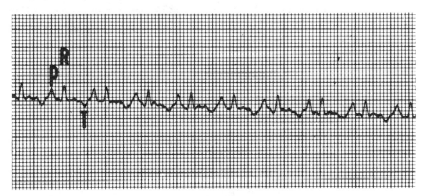

Figure 6–32 ▪ P pulmonale in the cat. In this lead II tracing, recorded from a 4-year-old male DSH cat with tricuspid regurgitation, the P wave is seen to be consistently taller than 0.2 mv (2 small boxes). (Paper speed = 50 mm/sec, 1 cm = 1 mv.)

II

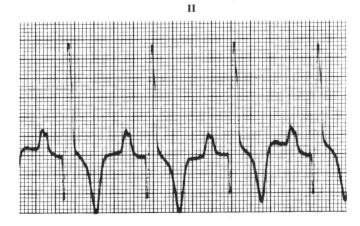

Figure 6–34 ▪ This lead II tracing demonstrates biatrial enlargement in a dog. The P waves are both too wide and too tall, and a notch can be seen at the apex. This recording was made at 50 mm/sec, with 1 cm = 1 mv, so the P wave is 0.06 sec wide and 0.5 to 0.6 mv tall. The electrocardiographic diagnosis is P mitrale and P pulmonale (biatrial enlargement). Left ventricular enlargement is also demonstrated by the wide QRS and S-T segment slurring. (From Edwards, NJ: Bolton's Handbook of Canine and Feline Electrocardiography, ed 2. Philadelphia, WB Saunders, 1987, with permission.)

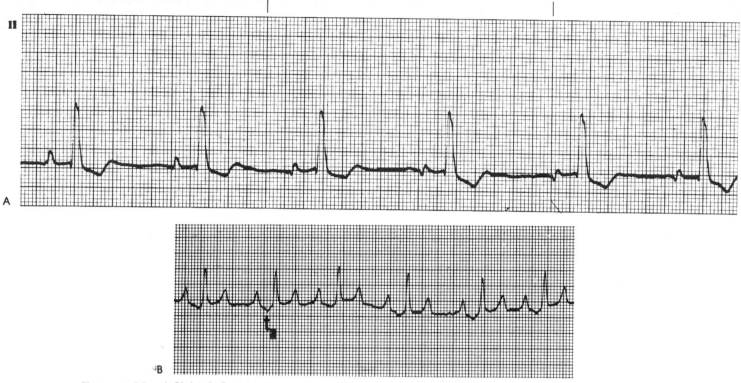

Figure 6–35 ▪ *A*, Biphasic P waves can be seen in the last four P-QRS-T sequences in this lead II ECG recorded from a dog. Note the first two P waves do not appear biphasic. As the pacemaker site shifts slightly, a different P wave configuration (biphasic P waves) can be seen. (Paper speed = 50 mm/sec, 1 cm = 1 mv.)

B, This lead II ECG was recorded from a 7-year-old mixed breed dog with heartworm disease. Note the consistent negative deflection in the P-R segment following each P wave. This is the T wave of atrial repolarization and is called an atrial T wave (T_A wave). (Modified from Edwards, NJ: Bolton's Handbook of Canine and Feline Electrocardiography, ed 2. Philadelphia, WB Saunders, 1987, with permission.)

DEFLECTION

The P wave is normally positive (above the baseline) in leads I, II, III, and aVF. In lead aVL it may be either positive or negative. In lead aVR it is usually negative (below the baseline). In the chest leads the normal P wave is positive in leads CV_5RL (V_1), CV_6LL (V_2), and CV_6LU (V_4) and is negative in V_{10} (V_6). In the base-apex lead utilized for the horse and cow, the P wave is usually positive. In general, the normal P-wave deflection should be in the same direction as the R wave in whatever lead you are examining, with the exception of the base-apex lead, in which the QRS is almost always negative.

OTHER IMPORTANT CONSIDERATIONS

1. P waves may be both too tall (P pulmonale) and too wide (P mitrale), suggesting enlargement of both the right and left atria.

2. P waves may occasionally appear biphasic — that is, part of their deflection is positive (above the baseline) and part is negative (below the baseline). The usual appearance of the biphasic P wave is an initial downward deflection followed by a positive deflection that leads into the P-R segment (Fig. 6–35A). Biphasic P waves are usually associated with a shifting pacemaker with a site that is outside the S-A node. Biphasic P waves as shown in Figure 6–35A should not be confused with atrial T waves (T_A waves). Atrial T waves are associated with increased current generated from atrial repolarization. They are usually seen as a negative deflection following the P wave and can be found within the P-R segment (Fig. 6–35B). Atrial T waves are often associated with right atrial enlargement.

3. Cats and toy breed dogs with left atrial enlargement frequently meet the criteria for P pulmonale before the P-wave duration exceeds 0.04 sec (P mitrale).

4. Intra-atrial conduction delays are not well recognized on the ECG and could contribute to an increase in height or width of the P wave without the presence of true atrial enlargement.

5. The shape and height of P waves may vary within any one particular ECG. If this variation is associated with a marked SA, it usually repeats itself periodically throughout the ECG associated with the phase of respiration. The polarity (direction above or below the baseline) should remain the same in any one lead. This is termed a wandering pacemaker (Fig. 6–36).

6. P-wave inversion in leads other than aVR (negative P waves in leads I, II, III, and aVF) may indicate that S-A node is not the pacemaker and retrograde (reverse) conduction is occurring throughout the atria. This is most commonly seen with disease states that result in an ectopic focus at or near the A-V nodal junction assuming the pacemaker role for one or more beats (Fig. 6–37).

7. P waves may appear to be absent or missing in some ECGs. If P waves cannot be found in the lead II rhythm strip, examine the other leads for the presence of P waves. If P waves are found in any of the other leads and the rate and rhythm in those leads are the same as those of the lead II rhythm strip being used for measurements, S-A nodal discharge, atrial depolarization, and conduction are in fact occurring. Why then are the P waves not visualized? Remember the ECG records the sum of the electrical activity on the body surface. In this case, that sum is at or near zero and no waveform is produced. This is particularly true for cats because their P wave is often difficult to see (Fig. 6–38). If P waves cannot be found in any lead, there is usually something wrong, frequently a supraventricular dysrhythmia of some type. Most often this is atrial flutter (Fig. 6–39), atrial fibrillation (Fig. 6–40), or sinoatrial standstill (Fig. 6–41). Note in all three of these examples there is an abnormality in the ventricular rhythm as well. If the ventricular rate and rhythm remain normal for the species being examined, even though you might not be able to visualize P waves they are probably still there. In this case, increase the sensitivity so that 1 cm = 0.5 mv (double sensitivity) and repeat the ECG recording in the hope of finding P waves (you are essentially doubling the size of all the waveforms). If that does not allow you to see P waves, record the chest leads and inspect them for P waves.

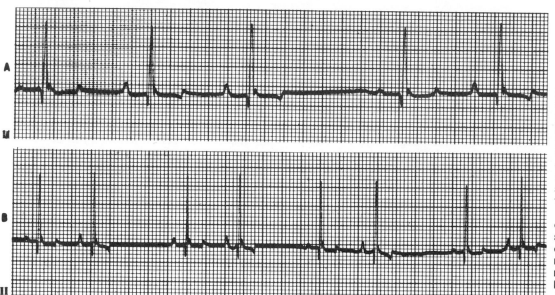

Figure 6–36 ▪ *A*, A more exaggerated sinus arrhythmia in a dog is shown. It is a sinus rhythm, and it is grossly irregular. If the pauses are measured, they are less than twice the normal R-R interval, which differentiates this from sinus arrest. *B*, The bottom tracing was recorded at 25 mm/sec to demonstrate that the rhythm is "regularly irregular." This is a clue that is associated with respirations, which are regular, and it is thus a hallmark of sinus arrhythmia. If the dog were watched, it would be seen that on inspiration two beats occur, and during expiration, the pauses occur.

This tracing also demonstrates wandering pacemaker. It can be seen that the P waves vary in height. They become smaller after the pauses, and larger as the heart rate accelerates. (*A* is recorded at paper speed = 50 mm/sec, 1 cm = 1 mv.; *B* is recorded at paper speed = 25 mm/sec, 1 cm = 1 mv.) (From Edwards, NJ: Bolton's Handbook of Canine and Feline Electrocardiography, ed 2. Philadelphia, WB Saunders, 1987, with permission.)

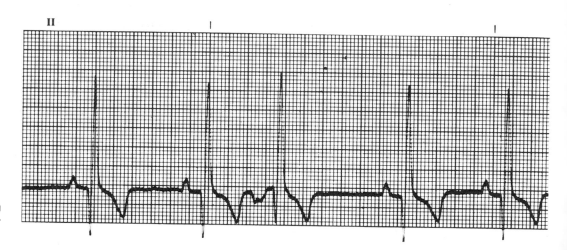

Figure 6–37 ▪ Nodal or junctional premature complex in a dog. (Courtesy of Dr. M. Lorenz.) Note the negative P' wave associated with this complex (third from the left).

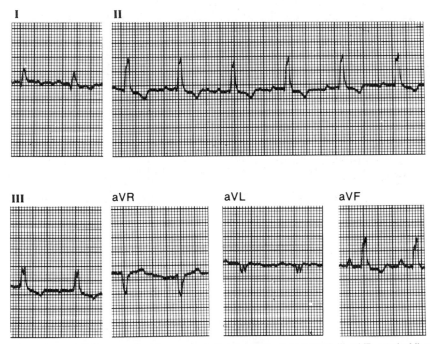

Figure 6 – 38 ■ Note in this ECG recorded from a cat, the P waves in lead I, II, III, aVR, and aVL are very small. If there was doubt about their presence and normal location, inspection of lead aVF confirms their existence and normal position in the P-QRS-T sequence. (From Edwards, NJ: Bolton's Handbook of Canine and Feline Electrocardiography, ed 2. Philadelphia, WB Saunders, 1987, with permission.)

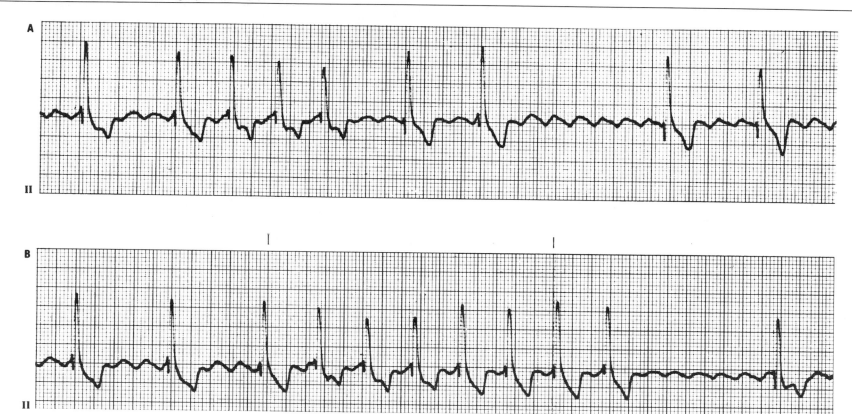

Figure 6–39 ▪ ECG diagnosis: atrial flutter. (From Edwards, NJ: Bolton's Handbook of Canine and Feline Electrocardiography, ed 2. Philadelphia, WB Saunders, 1987, with permission.)

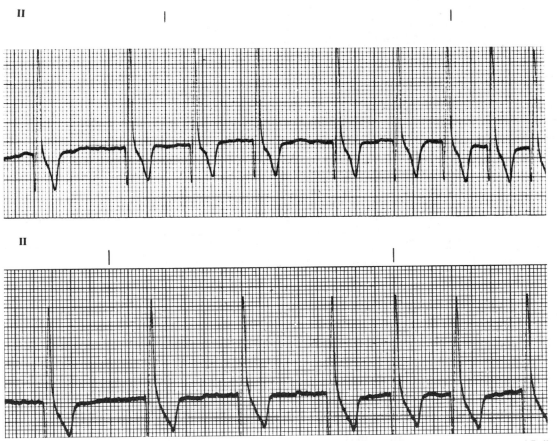

Figure 6–40 ▪ ECG diagnosis: atrial fibrillation. (From Edwards, NJ: Bolton's Handbook of Canine and Feline Electrocardiography, ed 2. Philadelphia, WB Saunders, 1987, with permission.)

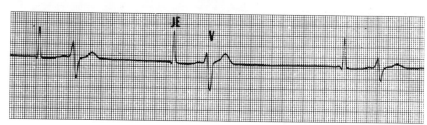

Figure 6–41 ▪ ECG diagnosis: sinoatrial standstill with junctional escape and VPCs. (From Edwards, NJ: Bolton's Handbook of Canine and Feline Electrocardiography, ed 2. Philadelphia, WB Saunders, 1987, with permission.)

TABLE 6–4 ▪ ECG Criteria for Atrial Enlargement

Electrocardiographic Features of Right Atrial Enlargement

1. P wave taller than 0.4 mv (dog) or 0.2 mv (cat)
2. Presence of t_a waves
3. P waves usually peaked rather than wide and rounded at their apex

Electrocardiographic Features of Left Atrial Enlargement

1. P wave longer than 0.04 sec in duration (dog and cat)
2. P wave may or may not be notched
3. Increase in width of the P wave may cause P-R interval to exceed its normal limits

Electrocardiographic Features of Biatrial Enlargement

1. P wave longer than 0.04 sec in duration (dog and cat)
2. P wave taller than 0.4 mv (dog) or 0.2 mv (cat)
3. Notching of the P wave is often present

*Modified from Edwards, NJ: Bolton's Handbook of Canine and Feline Electrocardiography, ed 2. Philadelphia, WB Saunders, 1987, pp 42, 45.

Significance of P Waves

The presence of normal P waves indicates that atrial depolarization and conduction have occurred and that the impulse originated in the S-A node. If there is a P wave consistently related to every QRS complex, the atrial impulses are being conducted to the ventricle. The size and shape of the lead II P waves can be used to assess the size of the right and left atria. The presence of abnormal P waves suggests atrial or junction dysrhythmias and/or atrial enlargement (Table 6–4). The absence of P waves in all leads suggests the presence of significant dysrhythmias. The identification, characterization, and measurement of P waves becomes the first and most important step in evaluating the ECG. In the horse, cow, sheep, goat, and llama, the shape and size of the P wave is not as important in assessing atrial enlargement as it is in the dog, cat, and ferret.

The assessment of P-wave existence and position in the normal P-QRS-T sequence remains very important for all species.

The P-R Interval (Fig. 6–42)

DESCRIPTION

The P-R interval represents the time during which atrial depolarization, A-V nodal, His bundle, bundle branch, and Purkinje fiber transmission of electrical activity are taking place. The P-R interval represents the electrical activity from the beginning of atrial depolarization to the beginning of ventricular depolarization (Fig. 6–43). The P-R interval is made up of the P wave and the P-R segment.

LOCATION

The P-R interval extends from the beginning of the P wave to the beginning of the QRS complex (see Fig. 6–1).

DURATION

The length of the P-R interval is determined by the width of the P wave and the rate of conduction of electrical impulses to the ventricu-

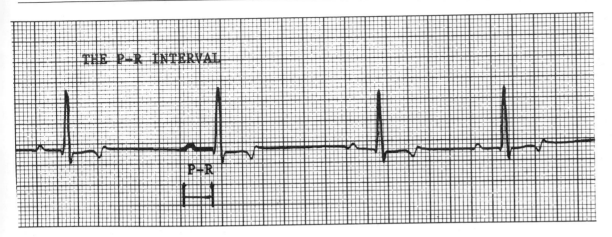

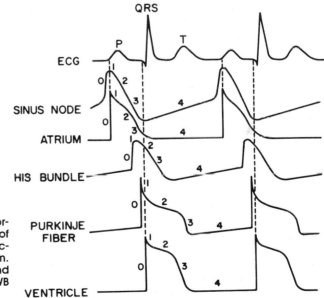

Figure 6–42 ■ The P-R interval is measured from the beginning of the P wave to the beginning of the QRS complex.

Figure 6–43 ■ The ECG is shown at the top, with corresponding action potentials of the different parts of the heart responsible for the production of the electrical current that becomes the electrocardiogram. (From Edwards, NJ: Bolton's Handbook of Canine and Feline Electrocardiography, ed 2. Philadelphia, WB Saunders, 1987, with permission.)

TABLE 6–5 ▪ Normal Values for the P-R Interval (Seconds)

Dog	0.06–0.13
Cat	0.05–0.09
Ferret	0.04–0.06
Horse	0.22–0.56
Cow	0.16–0.30

lar myocardium (length of the P-R segment). Table 6–5 summarizes the normal duration of the P-R interval for several species.

AMPLITUDE

The only amplitude the P-R interval has is associated with the P-wave portion discussed previously. No detectable waveform is produced on the ECG during the period of conduction through the A-V node, bundle of His, bundle branches, and Purkinje fibers. Consequently, the P-R segment becomes a flat baseline. Because the P-R interval is considered a measure of time, by definition, assessment of amplitude is not applicable to interpretation of the P-R interval.

CONFIGURATION

Because the P-R interval is a measure of time, assessment of configuration does not apply to interpretation of the P-R interval. One excep-

tion to this can be seen in Figure 6–35B, in which atrial T waves are seen during the P-R segment portion of the P-R interval. Atrial T waves (T_A waves) are associated with atrial repolarization and not impulse conduction through the A-V node, bundle of His, bundle branches, or Purkinje fibers; they merely occur at the same time and are visible during a period of otherwise negligible voltage formation.

DEFLECTION

Because the P-R interval is considered a measure of time, there is no deflection other than that produced by the P wave. Consequently, the evaluation of deflection is not applicable.

OTHER IMPORTANT CONSIDERATIONS

The duration of the P-R interval can be influenced by the duration of the P wave (width) or the duration of the P-R segment (length). Consequently, abnormal values for the P-R interval may result from either P wave or P-R segment portions.

SIGNIFICANCE

The P-R interval can provide evidence for conduction delay, conduction acceleration, and

continuity between atrial depolarization and ventricular depolarization. The assessment of the P-R interval is extremely important in evaluating the cardiac rhythm. Its length should be the same from complex to complex, because each P wave should be consistently related to its QRS complex. If the P-R interval is not a uniform length throughout the ECG tracing, an ectopic rhythm or a conduction disturbance should be suspected. Therefore, measurement of the P-R interval using either the "pencil-and-paper method" or the "caliper method" described for determining heart rhythm should be performed in several different sections of the ECG. The P-R interval should be the same in all leads of the ECG.

Prolongation (increase in duration or length) beyond normal indicates either enlargement of the left atria or delayed impulse conduction through the A-V node—usually the delayed impulse. Prolongation of the P-R interval is called first-degree A-V block (Figs. 6–44 and 6–45). Note that although the P-R interval is prolonged in these examples, there is a QRS complex that follows every P wave. This will become an important distinction between first-degree A-V block and the other types of A-V block when they are discussed in Chapter 7. The P-R interval can be prolonged by increases in vagal tone; extremely slow heart rate (bradycardia); atrial myocardial or A-V nodal disease; drugs that slow atrial and A-V nodal conduction, such as digitalis, beta blockers, and calcium blockers; antiarrhyth-

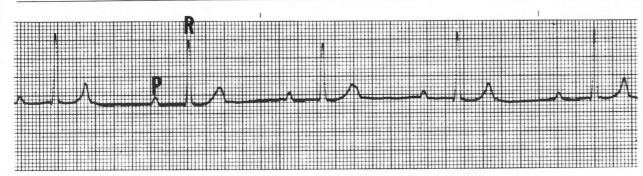

Figure 6–44 ▪ This tracing was recorded from a dog that was digitalis-toxic. First-degree atrioventricular heart block is present, because the P-R interval exceeds 0.13 sec. In this case it measures 0.18 sec. (From Edwards, NJ: Bolton's Handbook of Canine and Feline Electrocardiography, ed 2. Philadelphia, WB Saunders, 1987, with permission.)

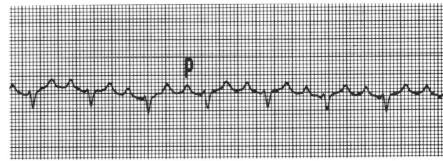

Figure 6–45 ▪ First-degree atrioventricular heart block in a cat is shown. The P-R interval exceeds 0.09 sec (in this case it measures 0.12 sec). (From Edwards, NJ: Bolton's Handbook of Canine and Feline Electrocardiography, ed 2. Philadelphia, WB Saunders, 1987, with permission.)

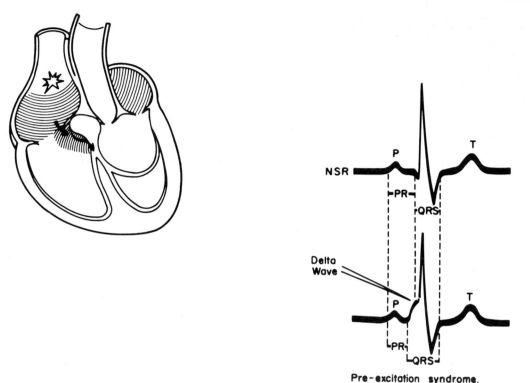

NSR

P

T

⊢PR⊣

⌐QRS⌐

Delta
Wave

P

T

⌐PR⌐

⌐QRS⌐

Pre-excitation syndrome.

Figure 6–46 ▪ Schematic representation of accessory pathway and conduction from the atria to the ventricles via an accessory pathway. (From Phillips, RE, and Feeney, MK: The Cardiac Rhythms. Philadelphia, WB Saunders, 1980.)

mic agents, such as quinidine, procainamide, and so on; and certain metabolic or toxic conditions, particularly those that result in hyperkalemia or endotoxemia.

Shortening of the P-R interval can occur with rapid heart rates (tachycardia), increases in sympathetic tone, beta agonist drugs, such as isoproterenol, dobutamine, and dopamine, or vagalytic drugs, such as atropine or glycopyrrolate. If an impulse originates outside of the SA node, particularly if the site of origin is near the A-V node, the P-R interval may be shortened. The most significant reason for shortening of the P-R interval involves the acceleration of impulse conduction completely, or partially around the A-V node resulting in a pre-excitation syndrome (Fig. 6–46). In these instances, the ECG will show a very short P-R interval. Often the ECG will look like the P wave blends directly into the QRS complex with no P-R segment being visible (Fig. 6–47).

The assessment of the P-R interval is an important part of electrocardiographic measurement, particularly as a sentinel for disturbances in A-V nodal conduction or dysrhythmias.

The QRS Complex (Fig. 6–48)

DESCRIPTION

The QRS complex represents ventricular depolarization. The QRS complex is usually the

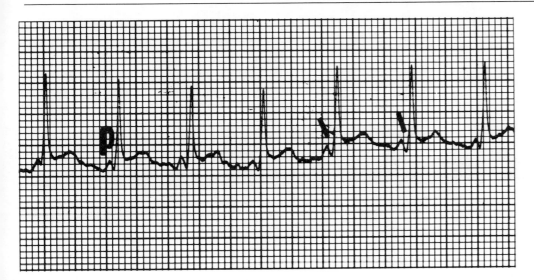

Figure 6–47 ■ This lead II ECG was recorded from a 4-month-old DSH cat with a ventricular septal defect. The P-R interval is shortened (0.03 sec) and the initial portion of the R wave appears to have a slight upward slurring in some complexes. Often this degree of slurring is very mild, and it is difficult to determine if the pre-excitation is of the Wolff-Parkinson-White (WPW) or Lown-Ganong-Levine (LGL) type. If the P-R interval is short and the QRS is of normal width, then LGL syndrome is the preferred diagnosis, as in this case. (From Edwards, NJ: Bolton's Handbook of Canine and Feline Electrocardiography, ed 2. Philadelphia, WB Saunders, 1987, with permission.)

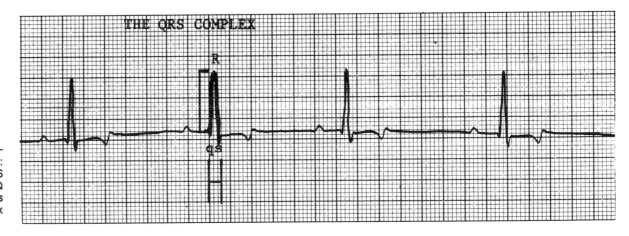

Figure 6–48 ■ The QRS complex represents ventricular depolarization and has two measurements: duration (width) and amplitude (height). The QRS duration is measured from the beginning of the Q wave to the end of the S wave. The QRS amplitude is measured from the top of the base line to the peak of the R wave.

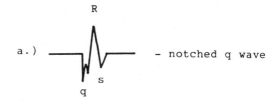

a.)   — notched q wave

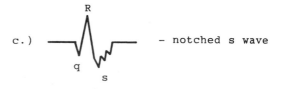

b.)   — notched R wave

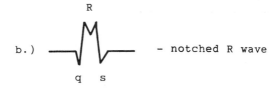

c.)   — notched s wave

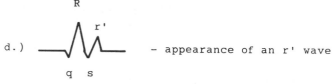

d.)   — appearance of an r' wave

Figure 6–49 ▪ Variations in QRS notching patterns are shown.

largest waveform of the ECG and may assume several different shapes. In any one lead, each QRS complex should look the same throughout the lead. If not, an abnormality is usually present. Notching of the QRS complex may also occur (Fig. 6–49).

LOCATION

The QRS complex follows the P-R interval.

DURATION

The duration (width) of the QRS complex is measured from the beginning of the first movement away from the baseline created by the P-R segment to the time the complex is complete and the S-T segment begins. When there are clear distinctions of the beginning and the end of the QRS complex, the measurement is relatively clear-cut (Fig. 6–50). Contrast this with the QRS complex in Figure 6–51.

When faced with the task of having to choose an imaginary spot to measure the endpoint of the QRS and the beginning of the S-T segment, it is sometimes helpful to use the baseline at the beginning of the QRS complex as a guideline. Using the level of this baseline, choose the spot at which the downslope of the R wave (as in the case of Fig. 6–51) crosses the level of the baseline and call that the end of the QRS complex. If an S wave is present, you would then select the point at which the up-

II

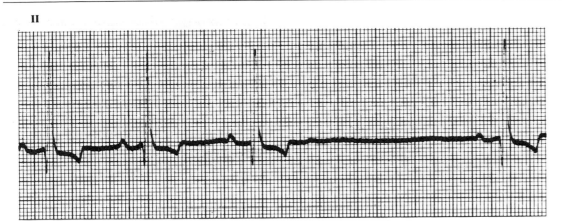

Figure 6-50 ■ Note the abrupt beginning of the q wave at the end of the P-R segment and the abrupt ending of the R wave at the baseline. No S wave is present in this ECG, making this a qR pattern for the QRS complex. The QRS complex duration here is 3 small boxes, or 0.06 sec. (Paper speed = 50 mm/sec, 1 cm = 1 mv.) (From Edwards, NJ: Bolton's Handbook of Canine and Feline Electrocardiography, ed 2. Philadelphia, WB Saunders, 1987, with permission.)

stroke of the S wave returned to the level of the baseline. The straight edge of a piece of paper placed across the QRS complex at the level of the beginning of the QRS complex will help to define this point. If there is a point where the QRS complex appears to end and it is not at the level of the baseline, choose the most obvious point of change and call that the end of the QRS complex (Fig. 6-52).

Normal values for the duration of the QRS complex are found in Table 6-6.

AMPLITUDE

The amplitude (height) of the QRS complex is measured from the top of the baseline at the

II

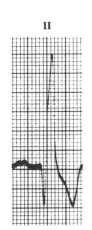

Figure 6-51 ■ In this lead II ECG tracing, it is difficult to pick an exact point where the QRS complex stops and the S-T segment begins. Note this is a qR pattern, as no S wave is present. To measure the duration (width) of this QRS complex accurately, it is best to pick the point at which the downslope of the R wave crosses the level of the baseline at the beginning of the Q wave. The QRS duration is 4 small boxes, or 0.08 sec. (Paper speed = 50 mm/sec, 1 cm = 1 mv.) (From Edwards, NJ: Bolton's Handbook of Canine and Feline Electrocardiography, ed 2. Philadelphia, WB Saunders, 1987, with permission.)

Figure 6-52 ■ In this lead II ECG tracing, the QRS complex has a qR pattern and the downslope of the R wave appears to change direction before it returns to the baseline, particularly in the third and fourth complexes. If the QRS duration was measured at the level of the baseline in this case, the measurement would be inaccurately wide. A more accurate measurement could be made by picking the spot above the baseline where the downslope of the R wave changes direction. The QRS duration here is 3½ small boxes, or 0.07 sec. (Paper speed = 50 mm/sec, 1 cm = 1 mv.) (From Edwards, NJ: Bolton's Handbook of Canine and Feline Electrocardiography, ed 2. Philadelphia, WB Saunders, 1987, with permission.)

II

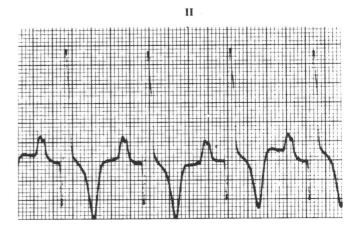

TABLE 6–6 ▪ Normal Values for the QRS Complex

	Duration	Amplitude
Dog (Toy Breed)	0.05 sec (max)*	2.5 mv (max)
Dog (Large Breed)	0.06 sec (max)	3.0 mv (max)
Cat	0.04 sec (max)	0.9 mv (max)
Ferret	0.04 sec (max)	2.5 mv (max)
Horse	0.08–0.17 sec	—
Cow	0.08–0.14 sec	—

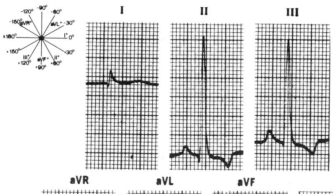

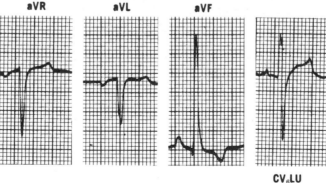

Figure 6–53 ▪ The amplitude (height) of the QRS complex in this ECG is 31 small boxes, or 3.1 mv. It is important to measure from the baseline and not from the bottom of the q wave. Remember, all measurements should be made in lead II. (Paper speed = 50 mm/sec, 1 cm = 1 mv.) (From Edwards, NJ: Bolton's Handbook of Canine and Feline Electrocardiography, ed 2. Philadelphia, WB Saunders, 1987, with permission.)

beginning of the QRS complex to the top of the R wave peak. Examine Figure 6–53 and determine the QRS amplitude. Remember, all measurements are made in lead II. Normal values for QRS amplitude are found in Table 6–6. Because of the penetration of Purkinje fibers throughout the ventricular myocardium in the horse and cow, the amplitude of the QRS complex in any one lead is not representative of cardiac size. Consequently, no normal values are listed.

CONFIGURATION

The QRS complex is comprised of three waveforms: the Q wave, which is the first negative wave following the P-R interval; the R wave, which is the first positive wave following the P-R interval; and the S wave, which is the first negative wave after the first positive wave (R wave) following the P-R interval. All three of these waves need not be present to create the QRS complex. Whatever combination is present should be considered as the QRS complex and measured as such. Review Figure 1–13 to better understand the possible combinations. A second positive deflection following the S wave would be designated an R' wave. A second negative wave following an R' wave would likewise be designated an S' wave. The largest wave of the QRS complex is identified with a capital letter (Q, R, or S) and the other components identified with lowercase letters (q, r, or s). The inscription must cross the baseline in order for a new wave to be formed. If it does not, the wave is said to be "notched" (see Fig. 6–49). Compare this with Figure 1–13.

DEFLECTION

The deflection of the portions of the QRS complex is determined by definition and discussed under "Configuration." In general, the QRS complex is positive in leads II, III, aVF, CV_6LL (V_2), and CV_6LU (V_4).

OTHER IMPORTANT CONSIDERATIONS

Increases in either duration (width) or amplitude (height) of the QRS complex beyond normal values usually indicate left ventricular enlargement. This may be dilatation or hypertrophy, or both. It is usually impossible to distinguish between the two on the surface ECG. The duration (width) of the QRS complex can also be prolonged by conduction delay in the left ventricle (complete left bundle branch block and left anterior fascicular block), by conduction delay in the right ventricle (right bundle branch block), or by severe right ventricular hypertrophy. In complete left bundle branch block the QRS complex duration is prolonged because of an increase in R-wave duration (Fig. 6–54), whereas in left anterior fascicular block and right bundle branch block it is prolonged as a result of an increase in S-wave

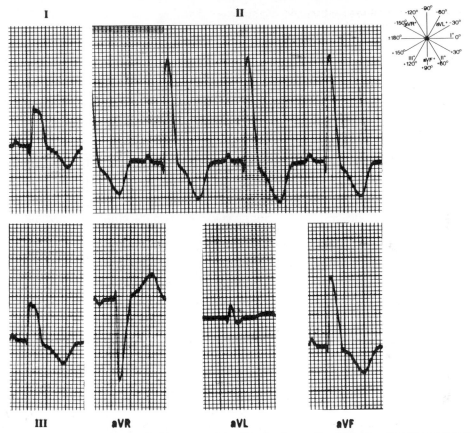

Figure 6–54 ■ This tracing was recorded from an older dog that was diagnosed as having endocarditis. Thoracic radiographs were not taken, but the ECG demonstrates a complete left bundle branch block pattern. The QRS complexes are large, wide, and positive in leads I, II, III, and aVF. Whenever the QRS complexes are wider than 0.07 sec (3½ boxes), left bundle branch block is diagnosed. These QRS complexes are 0.08 to 0.09 sec wide (4 to 4½ boxes). Complete left bundle block does not tend to deviate from the mean electrical axis, as does complete right bundle branch block. The mean electrical axis is +70° in this tracing. (Courtesy of Dr. J. Kazmierczak.)

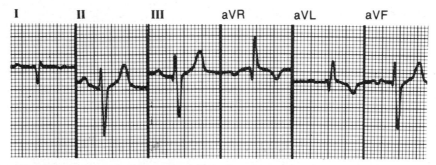

Figure 6–55 ▪ This ECG was recorded from a cat. Note the abnormally deep and wide S waves in leads II, III, and aVF. The finding of a Qr or qR pattern in leads I, aVR, and aVL, coupled with an rS pattern in leads II, III, and aVF, is consistent with a diagnosis of left anterior fascicular block. Note that the mean electrical axis is approximately −60°, another finding consistent with this diagnosis. (Paper speed = 50 mm/sec, 1 cm = 1 mv.) (From Edwards, NJ: Bolton's Handbook of Canine and Feline Electrocardiography, ed 2. Philadelphia, WB Saunders, 1987, with permission.)

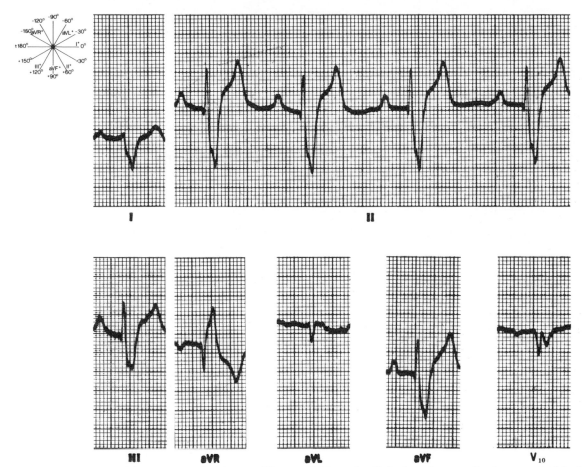

Figure 6–56 ▪ This ECG was recorded from a 10-year-old beagle. Note the abnormally deep and wide S waves in leads I, II, III, and aVF. Note also that the S waves have a notch in them and that almost all the width of the QRS complex is produced by the wide S wave. The findings of an rS pattern in leads I, II, III, and aVF and a qR pattern in lead aVR are consistent with a diagnosis of right bundle branch block. (From Edwards, NJ: Bolton's Handbook of Canine and Feline Electrocardiography, ed 2. Philadelphia, WB Saunders, 1987, with permission.)

width (Figs. 6–55 and 6–56). It is important, therefore, to determine which portion of the QRS complex is responsible for its total width being too great.

SIGNIFICANCE

Identifying and correctly interpreting the QRS complex is crucial to the assessment of ventricular health and to the recognition of arrhythmias. All QRS complexes within any one lead should look identical, and each one should be consistently related to the preceding P wave. If this is not the case, a dysrhythmia is present. Evaluation of the duration (width) and amplitude (height) of the QRS complex helps define ventricular size or conduction. Of all the waveforms, the QRS complex is the most important, as it represents the electrical stimulus for mechanical contraction (beating) of the ventricles. The QRS complex provides more information than any other waveform on the ECG.

The S-T Segment (Fig. 6–57)

DESCRIPTION

The S-T segment represents the end of ventricular depolarization and the beginning of ventricular repolarization. This is when the heart is completing the mechanical ejection

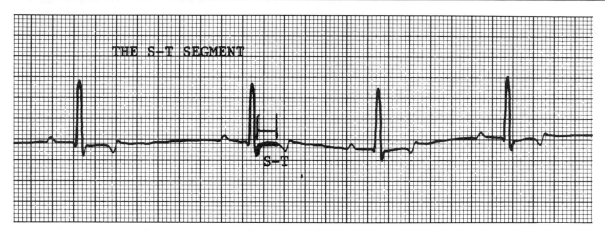

Figure 6–57 ▪ The S-T segment is measured from the end of the QRS complex to the beginning of the T wave.

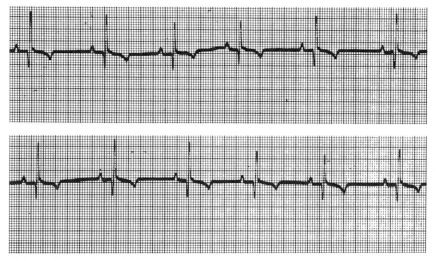

Figure 6–58 ▪ This continuous lead II ECG was recorded from a normal 2-year-old mixed breed dog. Note the period betwen the end of the QRS complex and beginning of the T wave. This is the S-T segment. It appears relatively flat at the level of the baseline and is clearly definable from both the QRS complex and the T wave. (From Edwards, NJ: Bolton's Handbook of Canine and Feline Electrocardiography, ed 2. Philadelphia, WB Saunders, 1987, with permission.)

of blood and is in the very early stages of relaxation.

LOCATION

The S-T segment extends from the end of the QRS complex to the beginning of the T wave. The point where the S-T segment begins and the QRS complex ends is called the "J point."

DURATION

Although the S-T segment represents a period of time during the P-QRS-T sequence, its duration is not usually measured as a distinct entity. It is included in the Q-T interval measurement.

AMPLITUDE

Under normal circumstances, the S-T segment remains at the baseline, as little net electrical activity is detected on the body surface during this period (Fig. 6–58). The S-T segment is assessed by its degree of elevation or depression from the baseline, which will be discussed under "Deflection."

CONFIGURATION

The S-T segment represents a measurement of time during the P-QRS-T sequence, and as

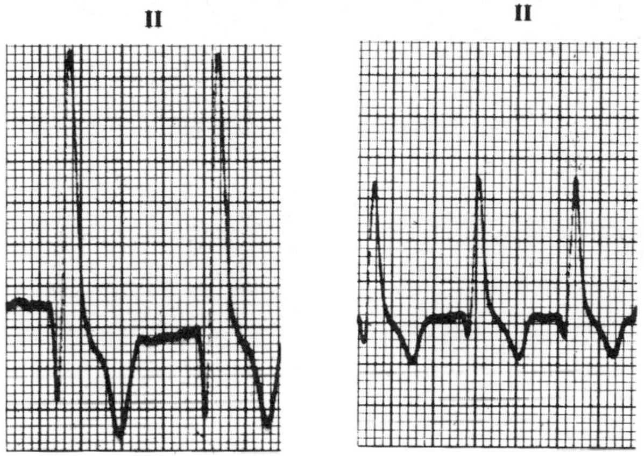

II   **II**

Figure 6–59 ▪ These two lead II ECG tracings were recorded from two different dogs. The S-T segment is not clearly discernible and appears to slide, or "slur," into the T wave. This is called S-T segment slurring and is commonly associated with left ventricular enlargement. (Paper speed = 50 mm/sec, 1 cm = 1 mv.) (From Edwards, NJ: Bolton's Handbook of Canine and Feline Electrocardiography, ed 2. Philadelphia, WB Saunders, 1987, with permission.)

such, assessment of configuration is not applicable. One exception is the presence of S-T segment slurring (Fig. 6–59). S-T segment slurring is seen when the S-T segment goes directly into the T wave without first straightening out even with the baseline. The presence of S-T segment slurring is often associated with left ventricular enlargement, frequently occurring in concert with wide QRS complexes.

DEFLECTION

The S-T segment is usually isoelectric, having the same position on the ECG tracing as the baseline. The normal S-T segment may be slightly elevated above the baseline or slightly depressed below the baseline. This amount of elevation or depression should not exceed two small boxes (0.2 mv) in the dog or one small box (0.1 mv) in the cat. Criteria for S-T segment elevation and depression in other species are not as well determined. However, any elevation or depression of the S-T segment in excess of two small boxes (0.2 mv) should be considered abnormal.

OTHER IMPORTANT CONSIDERATIONS

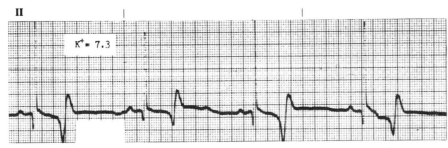

II

K^+ = 7.3

Figure 6–60 ▪ This lead II ECG tracing was recorded from a dog with Addison's disease. Serum potassium values were markedly elevated (7.3 mEq/liter). Note the S-T segment is about 10 small boxes (0.20 sec) long. (From Edwards, NJ: Bolton's Handbook of Canine and Feline Electrocardiography, ed 2. Philadelphia, WB Saunders, 1987, with permission.)

Electrolyte disturbances will sometimes cause changes in the S-T segment. Hyperkalemia or hypokalemia may cause prolongation of the S-T segment (Fig. 6–60). Hypercalcemia may

II

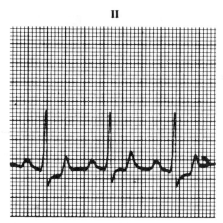

Figure 6–61 ▪ This lead II ECG tracing was recorded from a dog in respiratory distress. The S-T segment depression was thought to be due to myocardial hypoxia as it returned to normal after oxygen therapy. (From Edwards, NJ: Bolton's Handbook of Canine and Feline Electrocardiography, ed 2. Philadelphia, WB Saunders, 1987, with permission.)

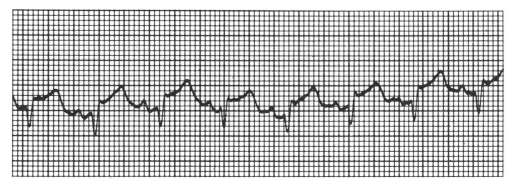

Figure 6–62 ▪ This lead II ECG was recorded on a severely dyspneic DSH cat with a diaphragmatic hernia. Note the negative rS pattern to the QRS complex and the marked S-T segment elevation associated with myocardial hypoxia. (Paper speed = 50 mm/sec, 1 cm = 1 mv.) (From Edwards, NJ: Bolton's Handbook of Canine and Feline Electrocardiography, ed 2. Philadelphia, WB Saunders, 1987, with permission.)

cause shortening and elevation of the S-T segment. Hypocalcemia may cause prolongation of the S-T segment. Pericardial effusion has also been associated with S-T segment elevation.

SIGNIFICANCE

A change in a patient's S-T segment, as S-T segment elevation or S-T segment depression of greater than 0.2 mv, is almost always associated with ventricular muscle abnormalities. Ventricular hypertrophy, myocarditis, myocardial hypoxia, myocardial ischemia, traumatic injury to the myocardium, pericardial disease, and disturbances in calcium metabolism have all been associated with S-T segment changes (Figs. 6–61, 6–62, and 6–63). Evaluate the S-T segment carefully, paying particular attention to its position above or below the baseline, and watch for the presence of slurring. Think of the S-T segment as a kind of barometer of "ventricular myocardial happiness."

The T Wave (Fig. 6–64)

DESCRIPTION

The T wave represents ventricular repolarization and, as such, signals the conclusion of ventricular ejection of blood, the completion of the

II

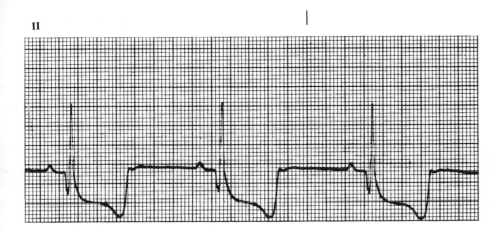

Figure 6–63 ▪ This lead II ECG tracing was recorded from a dog that had been recently hit by a car. Note the marked S-T segment depression associated with heart trauma suffered during the accident. This dog died within an hour after this ECG was recorded. An autopsy revealed severe bruising of the heart. (Paper speed = 50 mm/sec, 1 cm = 1 mv.) (From Edwards, NJ: Bolton's Handbook of Canine and Feline Electrocardiography, ed 2. Philadelphia, WB Saunders, 1987, with permission.)

Figure 6–64 ▪ The T wave represents the conclusion of ventricular repolarization. It has two measurements—duration (width) and amplitude (height). The duration is measured from the leading edge of the stylus line where it leaves the S-T segment baseline to the point where it returns and remains at the baseline. The amplitude is measured from the baseline to the peak of the T wave. Note that in this particular ECG the T wave is initially negative, then returns to cross the baseline, continuing to form a positive portion before returning and remaining at the baseline. This is a normal variation of the T wave and is called a biphasic T wave. When T waves are biphasic, they are usually measured for duration only and simply described as biphasic rather than calculating positive and negative amplitudes.

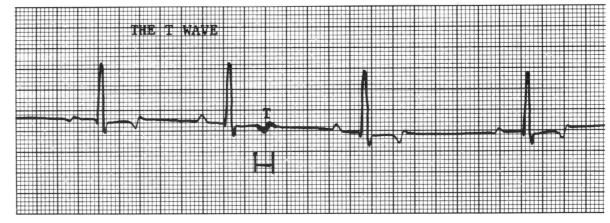

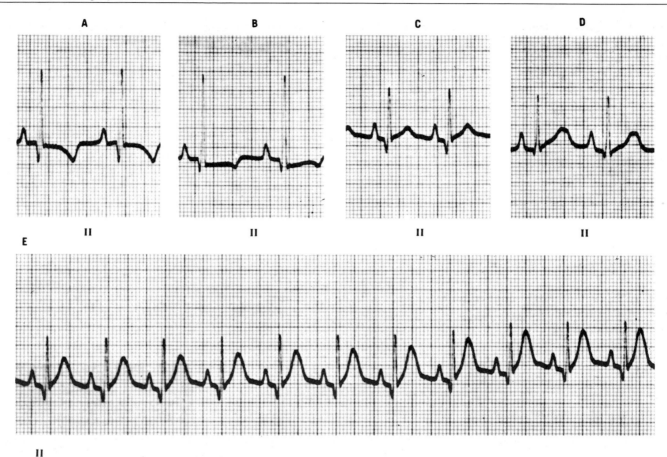

Figure 6–65 ▪ Note the effect of increasing myocardial hypoxia in this dog under anesthesia. All panels are lead II. *A* was recorded prior to the anesthetic procedure. During the anesthetic procedure (*B* through *E*) this patient became more and more hypoxic. Note the T-wave reversal that occurred at the time *C* was recorded. This was an early sign of myocardial hypoxia. Correction of the ventilation abnormality at this point would have avoided the sequence seen in *D* and *E*. Note the increase in heart rate, as well as T-wave and S-T segment changes in *E*. Failure to recognize these changes and correct the problem will result in arrhythmias and possibly cardiac arrest. (From Edwards, NJ: Bolton's Handbook of Canine and Feline Electrocardiography, ed 2. Philadelphia, WB Saunders, 1987, with permission.)

electrical events of the P-QRS-T sequence, and the impending diastolic rest period until the next S-A nodal discharge is formed.

LOCATION

The T wave begins at the end of the S-T segment and ends when its waveform returns to the baseline.

DURATION

The duration (width) of the T wave is measured from the end of the S-T segment to the point where the T wave returns and remains at the baseline. Although the T wave is routinely measured, no sound criteria have ever been established for its measurement in domestic species because of its extreme variability in normal animals.

AMPLITUDE

The amplitude of the T wave is measured from the top of the baseline to the top of the T wave. Criteria for exact T-wave amplitude measurements are not available for domestic animals. However, the T-wave amplitude is judged in relationship to the R-wave amplitude. In general, in lead II, the T wave should not be greater than 25 percent of the height of the R wave. If the R wave is not very tall, the T wave may

falsely appear too tall. As the ventricles enlarge, the QRS complex (R wave) and T wave generally enlarge proportionately.

CONFIGURATION

Very few restrictions are placed on the T wave in domestic animals. There are a few instances, however, where T-wave shape may be helpful in assessing the cardiac status of the patient.

Tall, broad, wide-based T waves are thought to be associated with myocardial hypoxia (Fig. 6–65). Tall, peaked T waves are often associated with hyperkalemia (Fig. 6–66); small, biphasic T waves are sometimes associated with hypokalemia. A change in T-wave configuration during an anesthetic procedure or over the course of a disease process, when compared with those in previously recorded ECGs, usually indicates myocardial hypoxia or ischemia (Fig. 6–65).

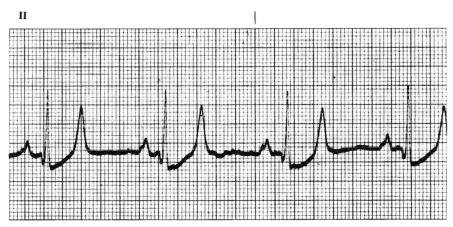

Figure 6–66 ▪ This lead II ECG was recorded from a diabetic ketoacidotic dog that was comatose. Note the tall peaked T waves consistent with the expected hyperkalemia of metabolic acidosis. (From Edwards, NJ: Bolton's Handbook of Canine and Feline Electrocardiography, ed 2. Philadelphia, WB Saunders, 1987, with permission.)

DEFLECTION

Normal T waves can be positive, negative, or biphasic in most leads. The T wave is normally negative in lead V^{10} (V^6), except in the Chihuahua dog. The T wave should be positive in lead CV_5RL (V_1).

OTHER IMPORTANT CONSIDERATIONS

Positive T waves in lead V_{10} (V_6) have been associated with right ventricular enlargement, usually hypertrophy in breeds other than the Chihuahua.

SIGNIFICANCE

The T wave represents the majority of repolarization of the ventricles and thus is an indicator of overall ventricular health. T waves signal the end of the P-QRS-T sequence. They may also contain "hidden" P waves when the heart rate is very rapid, as the next P wave is already being formed before the completion of the T wave of the previous complex. Slowing the heart rate will allow visualization of the normal T and P waves. T waves are affected most by ventricular hypertrophy, myocardial hypoxia, and electrolyte disturbances. The T wave should be closely scrutinized with regard

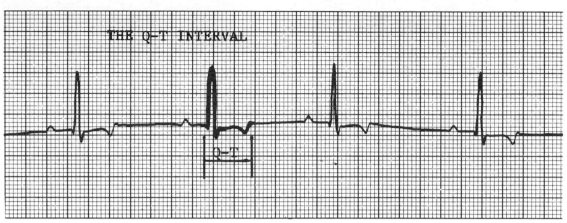

Figure 6 – 67 ▪ The Q-T interval is measured from the beginning of the QRS complex to the end of the T wave. It represents the total duration of ventricular depolarization and repolarization.

to its shape and size in relation to those of the R wave when evaluating the ECG.

The Q-T Interval (Fig. 6 – 67)

DESCRIPTION

The Q-T interval represents the period of time from the onset of ventricular depolarization to the completion of ventricular repolarization. The length of the Q-T interval varies inversely with the heart rate.

LOCATION

The Q-T interval extends from the beginning of the QRS complex to the end of the T wave.

DURATION

The normal values for the Q-T interval can be found in Table 6 – 7. The duration of the Q-T interval is inversely affected by patient heart rate: the faster the heart rate, the shorter the Q-T interval. Hypokalemia/hyperkalemia and hypocalcemia usually cause prolongation of

TABLE 6–7 ▪ Normal Values for Q-T Interval*

Dog	0.15–0.25 sec
Cat	0.12–0.18 sec
Ferret	0.10–0.18 sec
Horse	0.32–0.64 sec
Cow	0.32–0.64 sec

Note: Q-T intervals (in seconds) usually vary inversely with heart rates. Very rapid rates may shorten the Q-T interval below low-normal values. Very slow heart rates may lengthen the Q-T interval above high-normal values.

the Q-T interval. Hypercalcemia may cause shortening of the Q-T interval in some instances.

AMPLITUDE

Because the Q-T interval is a measure of time, assessment of its amplitude is not applicable.

CONFIGURATION

Within the Q-T interval are the QRS complex, S-T segment, and T wave. However, their shapes are not considered in the assessment of the Q-T interval. The sum of their durations, however, constitutes the Q-T interval.

DEFLECTION

Because the Q-T interval is a measure of time, assessment of its deflection is not applicable.

OTHER IMPORTANT CONSIDERATIONS

Drugs, particularly antiarrhythmic agents that cause prolongation of conduction or refractory periods, may cause an increase in the Q-T interval. Exercise or nervousness may cause artifactual shortening of the Q-T interval owing to their effect on sympathetic neurons that result in increased heart rates.

SIGNIFICANCE

The Q-T interval depicts the time needed for ventricular depolarization and repolarization to occur. Prolongation of the Q-T interval may indicate myocardial problems, toxicity, or hypoxia. As a general rule, the Q-T interval should be less than half the preceding R-R interval. Determination of the Q-T interval completes the standard measurement of the ECG. Although not as important as either P-wave or QRS-complex assessment, evaluation of the Q-T interval is important in having an appreciation of the overall electrical condition of the ventricles.

Application of Miscellaneous Criteria

The fifth and final step in the examination of the ECG is to review the tracing for miscellaneous criteria not observed in the first four steps discussed. These criteria are usually associated with right ventricular enlargement and include the presence of S waves in leads I, II, III, and aVF; deep S waves in lead CV_6LU (V_4); a positive T wave in lead V_{10} (V_6) in all breeds except the Chihuahua; and the presence of M- or W- shaped complexes in lead V_{10} (V_6).

S_1, S_2, S_3 PATTERN

In the dog, an S wave is not normally seen in lead I, is variable in lead II, and is often present in lead III. When all three leads contain an S wave, right ventricular enlargement usually exists. In the cat, S waves can be normal in all three standard limb leads. Consequently, the S_1, S_2, S_3 pattern is not a valid criterion for right ventricular enlargement in cats unless the depth of the S wave in all three leads exceeds 0.5 mv. An S wave is almost always present in lead aVF when the S_1, S_2, S_3 pattern is seen. S waves can be seen in leads II and III in normal ferrets. S-wave criteria for other species are not available.

DEEP S WAVE IN CV$_6$LL (V$_2$)

The presence of an S wave greater than 0.8 mv in lead CV$_6$LL (V$_2$) or greater than 0.7 mv in lead CV$_6$LU (V$_4$) is dependable evidence for right ventricular enlargement in the dog.

POSITIVE T WAVE IN LEAD V$_{10}$

The T wave in lead V$_{10}$ is usually negative. When it is positive, it is an indication of right ventricular enlargement in all breeds except the Chihuahua. The presence of M- or W-shaped complexes in lead V$_{10}$ may also occur in canine patients with right ventricular enlargement.

BIVENTRICULAR ENLARGEMENT

The presence of a wide QRS complex, deep Q waves, tall R waves, and a normal mean electrical axis usually implies biventricular enlargement. Frequently, S-T segment slurring, P pulmonale, or P mitrale may accompany these findings, indicating generalized enlargement of all four cardiac chambers.

DEEP Q WAVES IN LEADS I, II, III, AND aVF

Considerable disagreement exists as to whether the presence of Q waves greater than

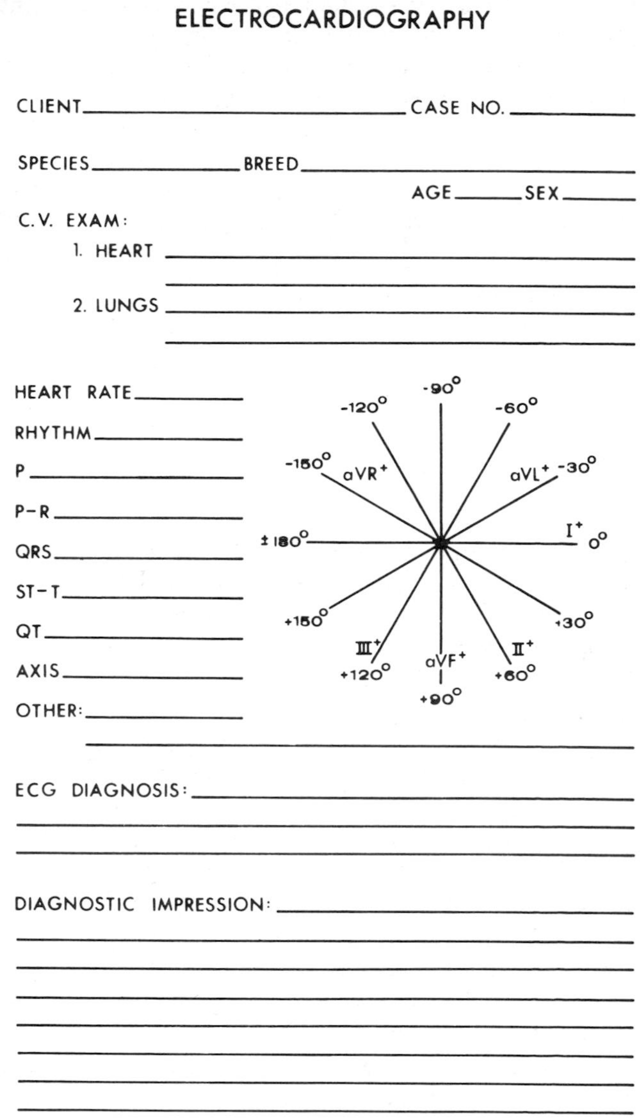

Figure 6–68 ▪ A form such as this one is designed for recording the electrocardiographic findings. Findings on physical examination may be recorded, and a case summary including chest x-ray findings may be written under "diagnostic impression." This form can be stored with the animal's record. (From Edwards, NJ: Bolton's Handbook of Canine and Feline Electrocardiography, ed 2. Philadelphia, WB Saunders, 1987, with permission.)

ELECTROCARDIOGRAPHY

CLIENT_____ CASE NO. _____

SPECIES_____ BREED_____
                                    AGE_____ SEX_____

C.V. EXAM:
   1. HEART _____

   2. LUNGS _____

HEART RATE_____
RHYTHM_____
P _____
P–R _____
QRS_____
ST–T_____
QT_____
AXIS_____
OTHER:_____

ECG DIAGNOSIS:_____

DIAGNOSTIC IMPRESSION: _____

0.5 mv in leads I, II, III, and aVF is a dependable sign of right ventricular enlargement. Some small breed dogs exhibit this ECG pattern when biventricular enlargement is present, but many normal larger breed dogs, especially those with deep chests, also show this pattern. Cats, however, rarely show this ECG pattern when the right ventricle is enlarged. Consequently, this criterion should be used with caution and should not be relied on unless other results (e.g., from ECG criteria, radiographs, echocardiograms) also suggest right ventricular enlargement.

RECORDING THE RESULTS

Once the ECG has been recorded and the measurements obtained, the results should become part of the permanent medical record (Fig. 6–68). When all five steps of the interpretation process have been completed and the results listed, an ECG-based diagnosis should be made and a treatment plan developed by the veterinary clinician–technician team. Subsequent electrocardiographic evaluations should be performed to assess the effectiveness of the therapeutic plan. Those results should also be recorded as part of the medical record. An updated problem list can then be developed and plans made for continued hospital care, patient discharge, and re-evaluation. It is vitally important that the veterinary technician be fully involved in all phases of this process. Refer to the section in Chapter 3 that discusses ECG storage and retrieval.

SELF-ASSESSMENT

After a detailed review of the process for electrocardiographic measurements, evaluate the ECGs in Figures 6–69, 6–70, 6–71, 6–72, 6–73, 6–74, and 6–75. Make all the measurements, following the five basic steps outlined in Table 6–1. For each ECG determine the following:

1. Heart rate
2. Rhythm
3. Mean electrical axis
4. Measure all waveforms (P wave, P-R interval, QRS complex, S-T segment, T wave, Q-T interval)
5. Miscellaneous criteria
6. Electrocardiographic diagnosis.

Compare your results with those listed in the Appendix (pp. 180, 181) for each of the seven ECGs. If needed, review the appropriate section of this chapter.

Every ECG that you see should be evaluated in this type of systematic manner. By doing so, you will become an invaluable part of the patient care team.

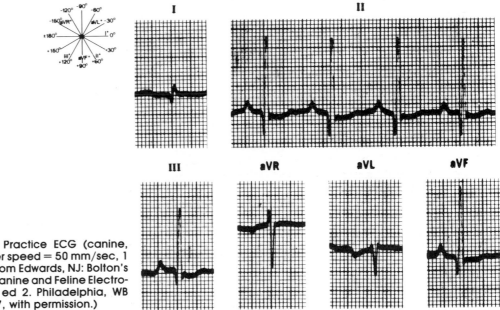

Figure 6–69 ▪ Practice ECG (canine, poodle). (Paper speed = 50 mm/sec, 1 cm = 1 mv.) (From Edwards, NJ: Bolton's Handbook of Canine and Feline Electrocardiography, ed 2. Philadelphia, WB Saunders, 1987, with permission.)

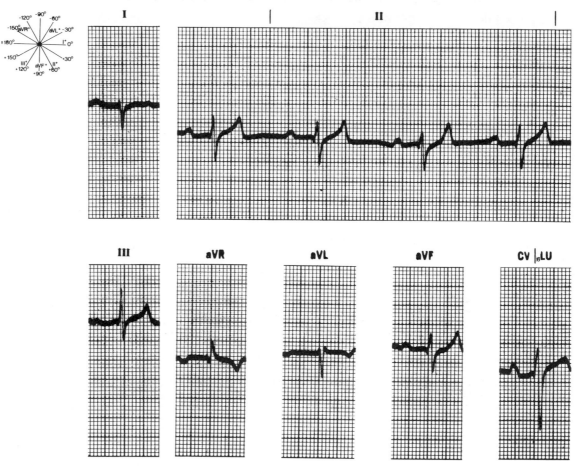

Figure 6–70 ▪ Practice ECG (canine, wire-haired fox terrier.) (Paper speed = 50 mm/sec, 1 cm = 1 mv.) (From Edwards, NJ: Bolton's Handbook of Canine and Feline Electrocardiography, ed 2. Philadelphia, WB Saunders, 1987, with permission.)

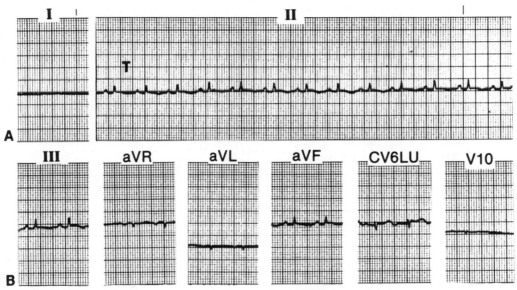

Figure 6–71 ▪ Practice ECG (feline, DSH). (Paper speed = 50 mm/sec, 1 cm = 1 mv.) (From Edwards, NJ: Bolton's Handbook of Canine and Feline Electrocardiography, ed 2. Philadelphia, WB Saunders, 1987, with permission.)

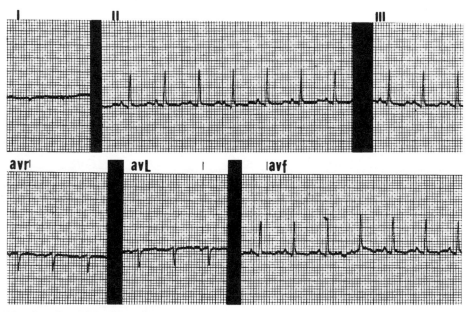

Figure 6–72 ▪ Practice ECG (feline, Siamese). (Paper speed = 50 mm/sec, 1 cm = 1 mv.) (From Edwards, NJ: Bolton's Handbook of Canine and Feline Electrocardiography, ed 2. Philadelphia, WB Saunders, 1987, with permission.)

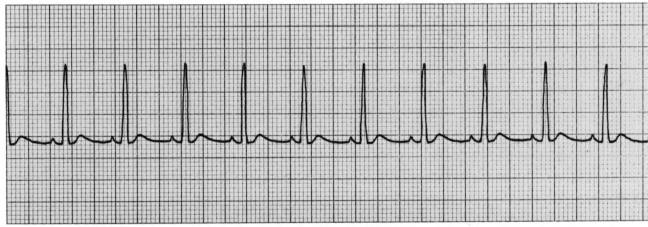

Figure 6-73 ▪ Practice ECG. This lead II ECG was recorded from a ferret. (Paper speed = 50 mm/sec, 1 cm = 1 mv.)

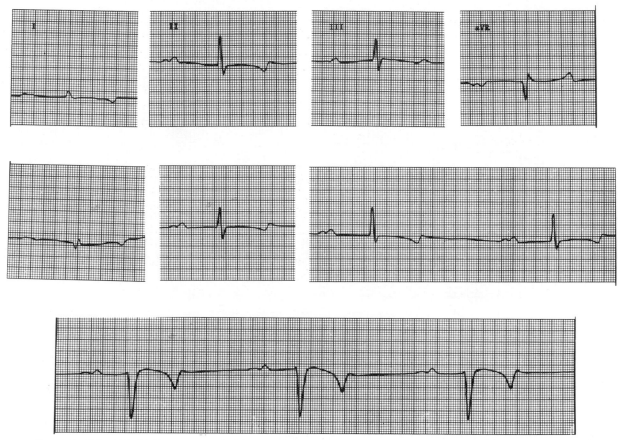

Figure 6–74 ▪ This ECG was recorded from a 20-year-old riding stable gelding. The middle section L → R is aVL, aVR, II; the lower strip is the base apex lead. (Paper speed = 50 mm/sec, 1 cm = 1 mv.)

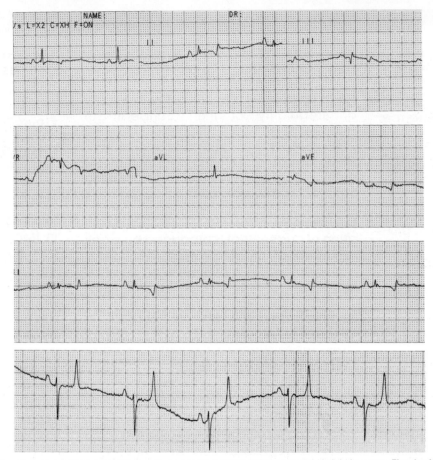

Figure 6–75 ▪ Practice ECG. This ECG was recorded from a 9-year-old Holstein cow. The bottom strip is the base-apex lead. (Paper speed = 25 mm/sec, 1 cm = 1 mv.)

P Wave The initial deflection on the ECG produced by depolarization of the atria.

P-R Interval Portion of the ECG measured from the beginning of the P wave to the beginning of the QRS complex.

P-R Segment Portion of the ECG measured from the end of the P wave to the beginning of the QRS comlex.

QRS Complex Portion of the ECG produced by depolarization of the ventricles. There are three main wavefronts: ventricular septal (Q wave), ventricular free walls (R wave), and ventricular and septal heart base area (S wave).

S-T Segment Portion of the ECG between the end of the QRS complex and the beginning of the T wave, that represents the initial slow portion of the ventricular repolarization.

T Wave The final deflection of the ECG produced by ventricular repolarization.

Q-T Interval The period of time from the beginning of the QRS complex to the end of the T wave; represents total time taken for ventricular depolarization and repolarization.

Heart Rate The number of times the heart beats per minute.

Heart Rhythm Description of the regularity or irregularity of the heartbeat sequence.

Mean Electrical Axis The direction of the main electrical force produced during ventricular depolarization.

Depolarization The discharge and generation of current that is produced by a cell or group of cells following the inward transmembrane movement of positive ions subsequent to an electrical stimulus.

Repolarization The return of the depolarized cell or group of cells to their resting state subsequent to the outward transmembrane movement of positive ions.

Hyperkalemia Elevated blood levels of potassium.

Hypokalemia Lower than normal blood levels of potassium.

Hypercalcemia Elevated blood levels of calcium.

Hypocalcemia Lower than normal blood levels of calcium.

Myocardial Hypoxia Relative lack of oxygen delivery or supply to the heart muscle.

Frontal Plane View depicting electrical activity (current flow) as "seen" from the patient's sternum; that is, right, left, cranial, or caudal.

Horizontal Plane View representing electrical activity (current flow) as "seen" from in front of the patient across the body, from right to left and sternal to spinal.

Transverse Plane View depicting electrical activity (current flow) as "seen" from the side of the patient; that is, cranial, caudal, ventral, or dorsal.

Bailey Six-Axis Reference System Arrangement of the bipolar limb leads (I, II, III) and the augmented unipolar limb leads (aVR, aVL, aVF) in a 360° circle in the frontal plane.

Dilation Enlargement of the heart caused by enlargement of the cardiac chambers.

Hypertrophy Enlargement of the heart caused by an increase in thickness of the myocardium.

Key Words Review

S-A Node The sinoatrial node, which is composed of special cells with fast rates of spontaneous depolarization, making it the normal cardiac pacemaker.

A-V Node The atrioventricular node, which slows atrial impulses as they enter the ventricle, thereby allowing time for the atria to empty before ventricular depolarization.

Bundle of His The portion of the specialized conduction system of the heart that connects the A-V node to the bundle branches.

Bundle Branches The right and left portions of the interventricular conduction system that terminate as the Purkinje fiber system.

Purkinje Fibers The terminal ramifications of the interventricular conduction system.

Right Bundle Branch Block Interruption of current flow along the right bundle branch of the interventricular conduction system.

Left Bundle Branch Block Interruption of current flow along the left bundle branch of the interventricular conduction system.

Left Anterior Fascicular Block Interruption of current flow along the anterior fascicle (portion) of the left bundle branch of the interventricular conduction system.

References

Blowers, MG, and Sims, RS: How to Read an ECG, ed 4. Medical Economics Books, 1988.

Conover, MB: Pocket Guide to Electrocardiography, ed 2. St. Louis, CV Mosby, 1990.

Conover, MB: Understanding Electrocardiography, ed 5. St. Louis, CV Mosby, 1988.

Edwards, NJ: Bolton's Handbook of Canine and Feline Electrocardiography, ed 2. Philadelphia, WB Saunders, 1987.

Fregin, GF: Cardiology in the Horse. Proceedings 6th Annual Equine Practice Seminar, New York State Veterinary Medical Society, 1982.

Kelly, WJ (ed): ECG Interpretation. Clinical Skillbuilders. Springhouse, PA, Springhouse Corp, 1990.

CHAPTER

7

Recognizing Abnormal Rhythms

The veterinary technician needs to be able to recognize life-threatening dysrhythmias. Because the veterinary technician is usually the individual recording the electrocardiogram (ECG), the first opportunity to recognize a problem belongs to the technician as the paper rolls out of the ECG machine. That is the best and perhaps only opportunity to begin the necessary response. The objective of this chapter is to enable the reader to make a rapid inspection of the ECG and, from that, a quick assessment of how serious the problem is and how rapidly it should be brought to the attention of the veterinarian. In order to appreciate the abnormal ECG, the veterinary technician must be thoroughly familiar with what is normal. It is hoped that the previous chapters have provided a basis upon which experience can be added to hone these important skills.

Although the height, width, and rate of ECG complexes vary markedly from patient to patient and species to species, the consistent relationship of the P-QRS-T sequence is common to all. This feature can be counted on to differentiate normal from abnormal. Obviously the electrocardiographic measurements are important in assessing the patient. However, these can usually be performed without risk at a later, more convenient moment.

Rhythm disturbances need to be recognized promptly. Recognition can be accomplished by determining the answers to the following basic questions:

1. Is the heart rate normal or abnormal?
2. Is the rhythm regular or irregular?
3. Can I identify P waves and QRS complexes?
4. Is there a P wave in front of every QRS complex and a QRS complex following every P wave?
5. Are the P waves and QRS complexes consistently related to each other (P-R intervals all the same)?
6. Do all the P waves look alike and do all the QRS complexes look alike?

Any artifact-free ECG recorded from any species can be evaluated rapidly using this simple technique. If the answer to any of these questions is "no", the ECG is probably abnormal. (Some variations will be discussed.) In general, the more "no" answers you have, the faster you should get help.

In reading this chapter, imagine that you are recording an ECG and what you are seeing looks like the ECG being discussed. Be sure that you understand the principles of evaluation and the physiologic basis of the ECG before proceeding.

Case 7 – 1 *(Fig. 7 – 1A):*

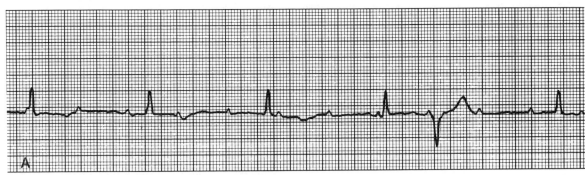

A

Figure 7 – 1 ■ A, Lead II ECG recorded from a male 18-year-old domestic short hair (DSH) cat. (Paper speed = 50 mm/sec, 1 cm = 1 mv.)

Questions

1. Is the heart rate normal or abnormal?
2. Is the rhythm regular or irregular?
3. Can I identify P waves and QRS complexes?
4. Is there a P wave in front of every QRS complex and a QRS complex following every P wave?
5. Are the P waves and QRS complexes consistently related to each other (P-R intervals all the same)?
6. Do all the P waves look alike and do all the QRS complexes look alike?

Discussion

Question 1. If you calculate the heart rate using the 1500 or 3000 method, by dividing the number of small boxes between R waves, the ventricular rate is 81 beats per minute. If you use the 10 or 20 method, the ventricular rate is estimated at 80 beats per minute. If you perform those same two calculations using the P waves, the atrial rate calculates as 188 and 200, respectively, for the same two methods. Consequently, the atrial rate would be normal for the cat, but the ventricular rate is much slower than normal for the cat. More importantly, we know the atrial and ventricular rate should always be the same. We must answer "no" to question 1. Something is happening to the electrical current of the P waves once they are formed.

Question 2. When either the caliper or the pencil-and-paper method is used, both the P-P interval and the R-R interval appear fairly reg-

ular. Note that there is an abnormal-appearing complex after the fourth R wave from the left, and that the fourth and fifth R waves are farther apart than we had expected, based on the interval between the previous R waves. Therefore, we can answer "yes," the atrial rhythm is regular but the ventricular rhythm is irregular.

Question 3. Were you able to identify P waves and QRS complexes? Some P waves are obvious in this ECG, but some may not be. What is the little bump at the very beginning of the first R wave? Using the paper-and-pencil method for marking P waves and shifting it backward (to the left) until the second mark lies even with the first readily seen P wave, you will find the first mark on your paper will line up directly on this bump. This should tell you to expect a P wave there, and in fact, the bump is a P wave hidden in the very beginning of the QRS complex (in this case, R wave) and can be easily identified. You should find five R waves plus the one abnormal-appearing complex between the fourth and fifth R wave. What is the positive deflection immediately preceding the abnormal-appearing QRS complex? Using the paper-and-pencil method again for identifying P waves, should a P wave be expected here? Yes, it should!

Question 4. Yes, there is a P wave in front of every QRS complex. But is there a QRS complex following every P wave? We must answer "no."

Question 5. If you measure the distance from the beginning of the P wave to the next nearest R wave, you will find there is no consistent value for the P-R interval. Again, the answer to this question must be "no."

Question 6. The P waves look alike when they are not hidden in the R waves! The QRS complexes do not all look alike owing to the abnormal-appearing complex between the fourth and fifth R wave.

To summarize, we have "no" answers to all or part of questions 1, 2, 4, 5, and 6. By visual inspection there are several important findings in this ECG:

1. The ventricular rate is much slower than the atrial rate.

2. No consistent relationship exists between the P waves and QRS complexes, suggesting they are in fact unrelated to each other.

3. One abnormal-appearing complex is present.

Let's discuss each of these separately.

The atrial and ventricular rate should always be the same in a normal ECG. Because the ventricular rate is much slower than the atrial rate (80 versus 188), something must be stopping (blocking) the electrical current from getting through the A-V node to depolarize the ventricles. (Review Chapters 1 and 6, if needed.) If some of the P waves were getting through the A-V node to depolarize the ventri-

cles, then these particular P-R intervals should be the same. In this case, none of the P-R intervals are the same, so none of the P waves are getting through the A-V node. This is called third-degree, or complete, A-V heart block and is usually associated with scar tissue formation in the A-V node, causing an electrical impasse. The abnormal-appearing complex between the fourth and fifth R waves is called a premature ventricular complex (PVC). You will see these also referred to as ventricular premature contractions (VPCs) or ventricular premature depolarizations (VPDs) in the medical literature. It is formed when an ectopic focus within the ventricular myocardium fires off before the normal firing sequence occurs (Review Fig. 6–43.)

Note the pause that follows it before the next R wave is seen. This is caused by a resetting of the "electrical readiness" of the ventricular myocardium to form the next R wave. PVCs are a sign of electrical irritability of the myocardium and usually indicate inflammation, infection, ischemia, hypoxia, infiltrative disease, or electrolyte imbalance.

The final ECG interpretation is third-degree, or complete, A-V heart block with PVCs and is often seen in aged animals with scar tissue formation in their hearts. These patients often show signs of lethargy, intolerance to exercise, weakness, or syncope (fainting). Their heart rates are invariably slow and are usually incapable of speeding up during exercise. See Figure 7–1B for labeling of the waves.

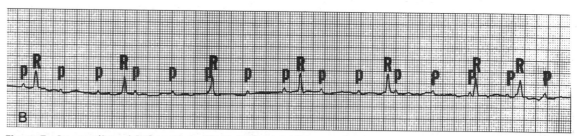

Figure 7 – 1 ▪ *continued.* B, Complete (third-degree) A-V block in the cat. Note the waveforms are labeled. No PVC is seen in this particular portion of the ECG, recorded on the same patient as in *A.* (Paper speed = 50 mm/sec, 1 cm = 1 mv.)

Case 7–2 *(Fig. 7–2):*

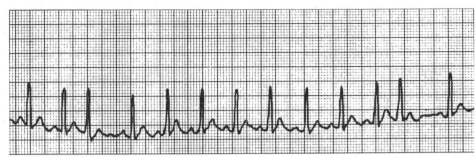

Figure 7–2 ▪ Lead II ECG recorded from a 4-year-old male ferret. (Paper speed = 50 mm/sec, 1 cm = 1 mv.)

Questions

1. Is the heart rate normal or abnormal?
2. Is the rhythm regular or irregular?
3. Can I identify P waves and QRS complexes?
4. Is there a P wave in front of every QRS complex and a QRS complex following every P wave?
5. Are the P waves and QRS complexes consistently related to each other (P-R intervals all the same)?
6. Do all the P waves look alike and do all the QRS complexes look alike?

Discussion

Question 1. If you used the 1500 or 3000 method the heart rate is approximately 250 beats per minute. If you used the 10 or 20 method the estimated heart rate is 240 beats per minute. This is a normal heart rate for the ferret.

Question 2. With either the paper-and-pencil or the caliper method, the rhythm is irregular in two places. Did you find them?

Question 3. Both P waves and QRS complexes are found.

Question 4. No P waves can be seen in front of the third and 12th complexes from the left. Note that there are two places where the rhythm is irregular. There does appear to be a QRS complex following every P wave. The small positive deflection between the T wave of the third QRS complex is a baseline artifact.

Question 5. When a P wave can be found, the distance between it and the succeeding QRS complex appears the same throughout the tracing.

Question 6. All of the identified P waves look reasonably the same. The third and 12th QRS complexes look slightly different than the remaining QRS complexes, which all look alike.

To summarize, we have "no" answers to all or part of questions 2, 4, and 6. By visual inspection the important findings in this ECG center on the P-QRS-T sequence associated with complexes 3 and 12.

Let's discuss these findings. In each of these complexes (3 and 12) we are unable to find P waves, the R-R interval with the previous R wave appears shorter than the most common R-R interval, and the R-R interval with the complex that follows complexes 3 and 12 is longer than the regular R-R interval. Thus, these complexes (3 and 12) are said to be "premature" (early) and are followed by a compensatory pause (delay) before the next P-QRS-T sequence is initiated. The shape of the QRS complex for complexes 3 and 12 is only slightly different than that associated with the normal P-QRS-T sequence. Because their shapes are only slightly different, there is good evidence to suggest that the electrical current generated in the atria traversed the A-V node and ventricular conduction system in a normal pattern. Where, then, are the P waves and why do the R-R intervals change on either side of complexes 3 and 12? The P waves are hidden in the T wave of the previous P-QRS-T sequence. They are hidden there because an irritated focus in one of the atria fired off early at the same time the T wave of ventricular repolarization was being formed. Because the atria fired early, the R-R interval with the previous sequence is shorter than normal. The prolonged R-R interval following complexes 3 and 12 is caused by a resetting of the "electrical readiness" of the atrial myocardium to generate the next P wave. Because the abnormal focus lies anatomically above the A-V node, it is considered supraventricular in origin. Complexes 3 and 12 are called premature supraventricular complexes or more commonly atrial premature complexes (APCs). The final ECG interpretation is APCs with evidence of P mitrale (wide P waves) and left ventricular enlargement (wide QRS complexes).

This ferret had dilative cardiomyopathy, and this ECG is typical of that condition. The ferret was also dyspneic, lethargic, and incapable of any exertion.

Case 7–3 *(Fig. 7–3A):*

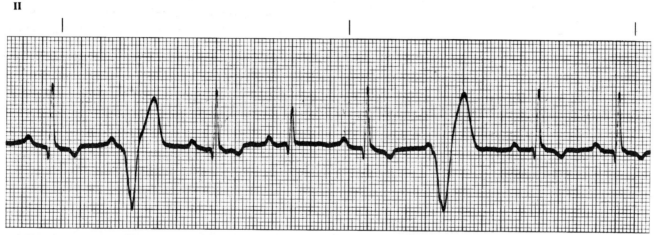

II

A

Figure 7–3 ▪ *A,* Lead II ECG recorded from a 10-year-old Great Dane. (Paper speed = 50 mm/sec, 1 cm = 1 mv.)

Questions

1. Is the heart rate normal or abnormal?
2. Is the rhythm regular or irregular?
3. Can I identify P waves and QRS complexes?
4. Is there a P wave in front of every QRS complex and a QRS complex following every P wave?
5. Are the P waves and QRS complexes consistently related to each other (P-R intervals all the same)?
6. Do all the P waves look alike and do all the QRS complexes look alike?

Discussion

Question 1. With the 1500 or 3000 method, the heart rate is approximately 150 beats per minute. With the 10 or 20 method, it is approximately 140 beats per minute. When using the 10 or 20 method all QRS complexes that fall between the hash marks should be counted, regardless of their shape. Either of the calculated heart rates is considered normal for this dog.

Question 2. With either the paper-and-pencil method or the caliper method, the rhythm appears very close to being regular.

Question 3. Yes, both P waves and QRS complexes can be seen.

Question 4. There is some question regarding the presence of a P wave in front of the second wide, aberrant (third from the right) complex. Using the paper-and-pencil method of marking P waves and sliding the paper, you will notice that a P wave would be expected close to where we see the small positive deflection immediately preceding the complex. Yes, there is a P wave for every QRS complex and a QRS complex for every P wave.

Question 5. No, the P wave preceding the second and sixth complexes is much closer to these complex than the other P waves are to their complexes.

Question 6. The P waves vary slightly in shape, particularly the one immediately preceding the sixth complex. All the QRS complexes do not look alike. Complexes 2 and 6 look the same but are unlike the rest. Complex 4 looks similar in shape but much shorter than its counterparts.

In summary, we have "no" answers to all or parts of questions 5 and 6. By visual interpretation the important findings in this ECG tracing are as follows:

1. The second and sixth QRS complexes look wide and bizarre.
2. The fourth QRS complex is considerably shorter than the rest.
3. There is slight variation in the shape of the P waves.

Let's discuss each of these. The second and sixth complexes are much wider and have a different shape than the rest of the QRS complexes. They look this way because they are the result of an ectopic focus firing from somewhere in the ventricular myocardium, causing the entire ventricle to depolarize. Because the path the electrical current took was not the normal one, the shape of the complex is abnormal. Because the path taken was from muscle cell to muscle cell rather than through the normal Purkinje system, the complex is much wider than normal. Although these complexes are not premature (note that they occur almost at the same time as an expected beat) they are from an ectopic ventricular focus and are called VPCs. When they do not disrupt the rhythm as in this case, they are called "mid" VPCs (Fig. 7–3B).

Complex 4 is called a "fusion beat." Note that its shape is similar but shorter than the normal QRS complex. A fusion beat or complex is formed when electrical current from the sinus node and electrical current from an ectopic ventricular focus meet somewhere in the ventricles. Think of it as though the appearance of the waveform is a combination of both the normal and abnormal patterns. The farther the normally conducted impulse gets into the ventricle before meeting the electrical

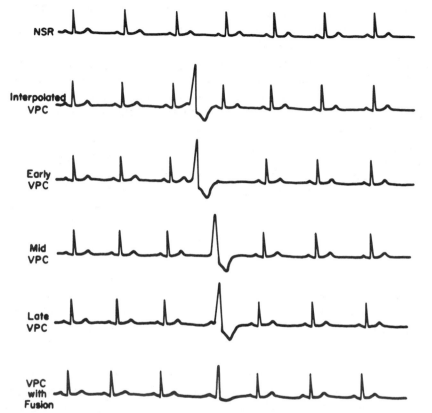

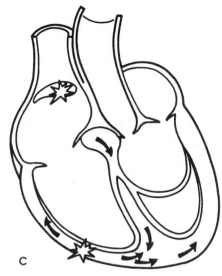

Figure 7–3 ▪ *continued. C,* Schematic representation of the simultaneous wave fronts of ventricular fusion originating from both the S-A node and the ventricular ectopic focus. (From Phillips, RE, and Feeney, MK: The Cardiac Rhythms. Philadelphia, WB Saunders, 1980, with permission.)

Figure 7–3 ▪ *continued. B,* Schematic representation of VPCs occurring at various times during the cardiac cycle. (From Phillips, RE, and Feeney, MK: The Cardiac Rhythms. Philadelphia, WB Saunders, 1980, with permission.)

wavefront of the ectopic focus, the more it will resemble the normal complex (Fig. 7–3C).

The slight variations in P-wave shape on this ECG are within the limits of normal. Technically this is called a wandering pacemaker, although the P-wave shapes usually vary more than these do with a typical wandering pacemaker. The minor shifting of the electrical wavefront is most influenced by vagal tone and is often correlated with inspiration and expiration in a repetitive manner throughout the ECG tracing.

The final ECG interpretation is VPCs with a fusion beat. This patient was severely anemic with a marked thrombocytopenia. Either the anemia, or thrombocytopenic bleeding within the myocardium could be responsible for this dysrhythmia.

Case 7–4 *(Fig. 7-4):*

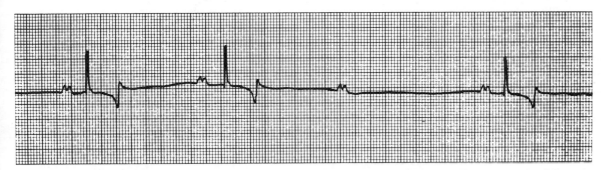

Figure 7–4 ■ This lead II ECG was recorded from a 6-year-old thoroughbred gelding. (Paper speed = 25 mm/sec, 1 cm = 1 mv.)

Questions

1. Is the heart rate normal or abnormal?
2. Is the rhythm regular or irregular?
3. Can I identify P waves and QRS complexes?
4. Is there a P wave in front of every QRS complex and a QRS complex following every P wave?
5. Are the P waves and QRS complexes consistently related to each other? (P-R intervals all the same)
6. Do all the P waves look alike and do all the QRS complexes look alike?

Discussion

Question 1. With the 1500 or 3000 method the atrial rate is 31 to 33 per minute. A quick assessment using the 10 or 20 method indicates the atrial rate is approximately 30 beats per minute. What is the ventricular rate? Because of the large variation in R-R intervals, the 10 or 20 method is preferred over the 1500 or 3000 method. An estimate of 20 beats per minute would be close in this instance. Remember, this ECG was recorded at 25 mm/sec paper speed.

Question 2. Visual inspection reveals an irregular rhythm when the R-R intervals are examined. Yet when the P-P intervals are assessed, using either the caliper or paper-and-pencil method, they appear almost regular.

Question 3. Both P waves and QRS complexes can be identified. The P waves have the notched appearance typical of the equine P wave.

Question 4. Each of the three QRS complexes (qR complex in this case) has a P wave preceding it, but the third P wave from the left does not have a QRS complex following it.

Question 5. Close observation and measurement of the P-R intervals reveals the first and last P-R interval are the same (8 small boxes, or 0.32 sec). However, the second P-R interval measures 9 small boxes or 0.36 sec in duration. Because the third P wave has no QRS complex following it, no P-R interval can be calculated.

Question 6. All four of the P waves do look alike, as do all three QRS complexes.

To summarize, we have an irregular ventricular rate with more P waves than QRS complexes and an absence of a QRS complex following the third P wave. The P-R intervals are not all the same, with the one that was different (longer in this case) happening in the P-QRS-T sequence preceding the P wave that has no QRS following it.

The electrocardiographic diagnosis in this case is second-degree A-V heart block. Note the third P wave was initiated at the predictable time, but the impulse never made it to the ventricles to cause the formation of a QRS complex. Because this P wave (the third one) looks exactly like the other P waves, we can safely assume the electrical impulse went all the way through the atria without any trouble but could not get through the A-V node to depolarize the ventricles. Hence, the term "A-V block." It is called second-degree A-V block because some of the other P waves (all of the others in this case) were able to get through and depolarize the ventricles. If the P waves are delayed beyond the normal range (0.22 to 0.56 sec in the horse) yet they all get through to depolarize the ventricle, then first-degree A-V heart block is said to be present. If no P waves are able to get through to depolarize the ventri-

cles, and the ventricles consequently begin beating on their own, then third-degree, or complete, A-V block is present. In this case of second-degree block, the prolongation of the P-R interval preceding the blocked P wave is significant. It is an indication that during this P-QRS-T sequence (the second one), the P wave had some difficulty getting through but did make it, even though it took longer than expected. This pattern is almost always due to increased levels of influence of the vagus nerve on the A-V node (increased vagal tone), resulting in slowing or stopping of electrical conduc-

tion through the A-V node. This is also called Mobitz type I A-V block or Wenckebach A-V block. In the resting horse this is a "normal" abnormality because of the high vagal tone present in the horse, and it almost always disappears when the horse is exercised. If you see this type of second-degree A-V block in the horse you should exercise the horse for 5 to 10 minutes and immediately repeat the ECG. It is only when second-degree A-V block persists following exercise that this dysrhythmia should be considered abnormal in the horse.

Case 7–5 *(Fig. 7–5):*

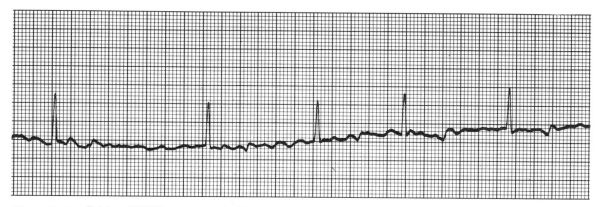

Figure 7–5 ▪ This lead II ECG was recorded from a 4-year-old Holstein cow with a left abomasal displacement. (Paper speed = 25 mm/sec, 1 cm = 1 mv.)

Questions

1. Is the heart rate normal or abnormal?
2. Is the rhythm regular or irregular?
3. Can I identify P waves and QRS complexes?
4. Is there a P wave in front of every QRS complex and a QRS complex following every P wave?
5. Are the P waves and QRS complexes consistently related to each other (P-R intervals all the same)?
6. Do all the P waves look alike and do all the QRS complexes look alike?

Discussion

Question 1. Because of the irregularity of the R-R interval, the 10 or 20 method is preferred to assess the heart rate rapidly. In this case the heart rate is approximately 100 beats per minute, or twice the top normal value for the cow.

Question 2. The rhythm appears irregular, as there is considerable variation in the R-R interval.

Question 3. There are five QRS complexes seen in this ECG but no definite P waves are seen. Instead we have a wavy baseline that looks like it might be one P wave right after the other, even in the baseline immediately after the QRS complex.

Question 4. Because we cannot identify P waves, we cannot say there is a P wave for every QRS and a QRS for every P wave.

Question 5. Because we are unable to identify P waves, we cannot assess the P-R interval.

Question 6. All of the QRS complexes look basically alike. However, because we cannot detect P waves we are unable to say whether they are alike or not.

To summarize, we have answered "no" to all or parts of questions 1, 2, 3, 4, 5, and 6. The key finding in this ECG is the inability to identify P waves. In addition, other abnormalities include an undulating wavy baseline that does not become isoelectric (flat), an irregular R-R interval, and a ventricular rate that is too fast for the cow. These findings are hallmarks of the dysrhythmia of atrial fibrillation.

Atrial fibrillation, commonly referred to as "atrial fib," is a result of chaotic, unorganized atrial impulses or wavelets of electrical activity called "f waves" that form in the atrial myocardium and take the place of the normal P wave. They bombard the A-V node with many random impulses, some of which get conducted to the ventricles, which causes an irregular ventricular rhythm that is almost always faster than the normal sinus rhythm of the species. Although irregular and rapid, the QRS complexes are usually of normal or near-normal configuration (shape) unless the ventricular myocardium or conduction system is also abnormal.

In the cow, atrial fibrillation is often seen in conjunction with disorders of the digestive tract and usually occurs secondary to changes in vagal tone rather than occurring as primary heart disease. Correction of the digestive tract disorder may result in spontaneous conversion to a normal rhythm or specific treatment for the atrial fibrillation may be required.

Case 7-6 *(Fig. 7-6):*

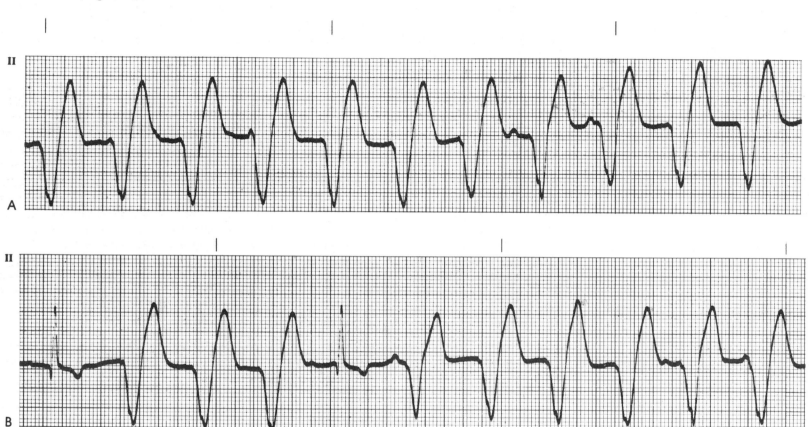

Figure 7-6 ▪ This continuous lead II ECG was recorded from a Great Dane dog. (Paper speed = 50 mm/sec, 1 cm = 1 mv.) (From Edwards, NJ: Bolton's Handbook of Canine and Feline Electrocardiography, ed 2. Philadelphia, WB Saunders, 1987, with permission.)

Questions

1. Is the heart rate normal or abnormal?
2. Is the rhythm regular or irregular?
3. Can I identify P waves and QRS complexes?
4. Is there a P wave in front of every QRS complex and a QRS complex following every P wave?
5. Are the P waves and QRS complexes consistently related to each other (P-R intervals all the same)?
6. Do all the P waves look alike and do all the QRS complexes look alike?

Discussion

Question 1. With the 1500 or 3000 method, the heart rate is approximately 158 beats per minute. With the 10 or 20 method, it is calculated at approximately 155, which is within the limits of normal for the dog.

Question 2. Either the paper-and-pencil or the calipers method shows a relatively regular rhythm.

Question 3. P waves are hard to find. There are occasional spots where positive deflections resembling P waves can be seen (in front of the fourth, eighth, and ninth complexes). In the lower strip only two normal-appearing QRS complexes are seen (first and fifth complexes). The remainder are bizarre.

Question 4. We cannot find a P wave in front of every QRS complex nor can we be sure that a QRS complex follows every P wave, as we have difficulty finding the P waves.

Question 5. There is no consistent relationship between what we are calling P waves and the QRS complexes.

Question 6. The P waves that were identified all look very similar but the QRS complex assumes various shapes and sizes.

In summary, we have "no" answers to all or part of questions 4, 5, and 6. By visual inspection, the important findings in this ECG are:

1. It is hard to find P waves.
2. All of the QRS complexes with the exception of the first and fifth complexes in the lower strip have a bizarre appearance. None of the abnormal QRS complexes have P waves consistently related to them.

Let's discuss each of these. The reason it is difficult to find P waves is that they are buried (hidden) in the abnormal QRS complexes. Only occasionally do they sneak out and become visible. If you use the paper-and-pencil method and mark the two P waves in the upper tracing, it is possible to get a rough idea of where the P waves might fall and an appreciation for why they are not visible.

The bizarre wide QRS complexes are all VPCs. They are abnormal and not associated with P waves. The presence of four or more VPCs in succession is called "ventricular tachycardia." The two normal-appearing QRS complexes are called "capture beats." Their P waves (not clearly visible) happened to fire at exactly the right moment to be conducted to and through the ventricles, producing a normal complex. The presence of these capture beats tells us that the others are all abnormal and meet the criteria for ventricular tachycardia.

The final ECG interpretation is multiform ventricular tachycardia with capture beats. Because the shape of the VPCs is not uniform, the term "multiform" is used to describe this type of ventricular tachycardia ("V tach"). If they looked exactly the same, the term "uniform" would be used.

This serious dysrhythmia should be brought to the clinician's attention immediately. Untreated, this rhythm can deteriorate rapidly into a life-threatening state. Intravenous (IV) lidocaine as an initial bolus followed by a constant-rate IV infusion of lidocaine is considered the treatment of choice.

Case 7–7 *(Fig. 7–7):*

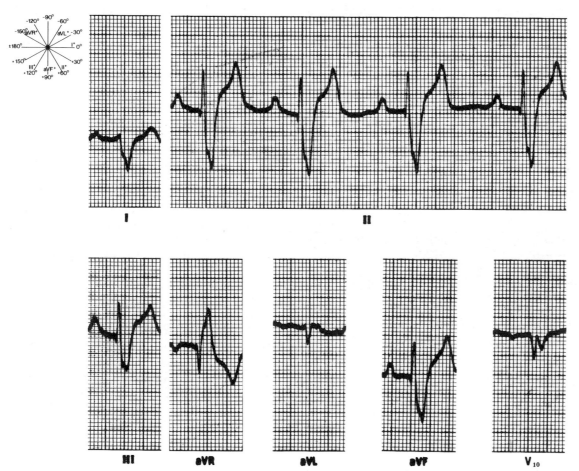

Figure 7–7 ▪ This ECG was recorded from a 10-year-old beagle. (From Edwards, NJ: Bolton's Handbook of Canine and Feline Electrocardiography, ed 2. Philadelphia, WB Saunders, 1987, with permission.)

Questions

1. Is the heart rate normal or abnormal?
2. Is the rhythm regular or irregular?
3. Can I identify P waves and QRS complexes?
4. Is there a P wave in front of every QRS complex and a QRS complex following every P wave?
5. Are the P waves and QRS complexes consistently related to each other? (P-R intervals all the same)
6. Do all the P waves look alike and do all the QRS complexes look alike?

Discussion

Question 1. Because no hash marks are evident on this tracing, the 10 or 20 method cannot be used. Calculating the heart rate by the 1500 or 3000 method indicates the rate to be 107 beats per minute, which is normal for the dog.

Question 2. Both the atrial and ventricular rhythms appear regular.

Question 3. P waves and QRS complexes can be identified.

Question 4. Each QRS complex has a P wave in front of it and each P wave is followed by a QRS complex.

Question 5. The P waves and QRS complexes appear to be regularly related to each other.

Question 6. Yes, all the P waves look the same and all the QRS complexes look the same.

In summary, we have answered "yes" to all the questions; there are no "no" answers. By visual inspection, however, the QRS complexes appear bizarre and somewhat like VPCs. Why then are there no "no" answers? The key here is the fact that there is a definite relationship within the P-QRS-T sequence.

The abnormality is in the conduction of electrical activity through the ventricular conduction system not in the generation of a ventricular myocardial impulse outside the conduction system. Note the initial portion of the QRS complex begins normally with a very small q wave and an r wave of normal width. It is the wide, deep, irregular S wave that makes the complex look abnormal.

The final ECG interpretation is right bundle branch block. This dysrhythmia is generally not detrimental to the mechanical performance of the heart and does not require treatment per se.

Case 7–8 *(Fig. 7–8):*

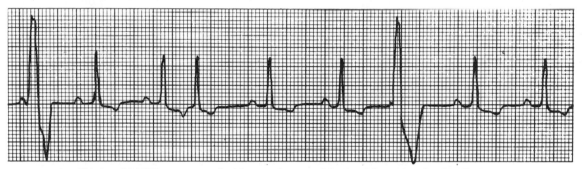

Figure 7–8 ▪ This lead II ECG was recorded from a 2-year-old mixed breed male dog that had been hit by a car 48 hours before. (Paper speed = 50 mm/sec, 1 cm = 1 mv.)

Questions

1. Is the heart rate normal or abnormal?
2. Is the rhythm regular or irregular?
3. Can I identify P waves and QRS complexes?
4. Is there a P wave in front of every QRS complex and a QRS complex following every P wave?
5. Are the P waves and QRS complexes consistently related to each other (P-R intervals all the same)?
6. Do all the P waves look alike and do all the QRS complexes look alike?

Discussion

Question 1. The R-R interval between normal P-QRS-T units is 19 small boxes. If you divided 3000 by 19, the heart rate would be 158 beats per minute, which is a normal rate for the dog.

Question 2. The rhythm is irregular by visual inspection, paper-and-pencil method, or caliper method.

Question 3. Yes, there are P waves and QRS complexes.

Question 4. No, the fourth complex from the left does not appear to have a P wave in front of the QRS. On close inspection, you will see two bizarre complexes. The second one, third from the end, has a tiny positive wave immediately in front of the complex. Is it a P wave? If you check the P-P interval using either the paper-and-pencil method or the caliper method, you will see a P wave would be expected just about where this tiny blip is. Therefore, this little blip is probably the beginning of a P wave. All of the P waves appear to be followed by a QRS complex.

Question 5. No. The first P wave occurs shortly before the bizarre complex. The second, third, fifth, sixth, eighth, and ninth P-R intervals all appear the same. The second bizarre complex also has a P wave occurring just as the bizarre complex begins.

Question 6. No. The P wave associated with the second bizarre QRS does not look like the rest. Two bizarre QRS complexes (1 and 7) appear much different from the rest. Also, look carefully at the T wave of the third complex from the left and compare it with the other T waves. What do you see? This T wave is slightly narrower than the others and slightly more negative than the others. Why? Is this artifact? Note the closeness of the fourth QRS complex to the third (short R-R interval), compared with the rest of the ECG. Also note that both of these QRS complexes look alike. The fourth one is a premature supraventricular complex whose P wave is hidden in the T wave of the third P-QRS-T sequence; hence, the slightly different shape of the third T wave. Because it is more negative, we can assume that the focus responsible for the premature supraventricular complex is in the lower portion of the atria, and retrograde (backward) atrial conduction is occurring from this site toward the S-A node, producing a negative voltage and hence a negative P wave. These are more specifically called junctional premature complexes. The reason the resulting R wave looks normal is that the A-V nodal and ventricular conduction are normal. Note also the pause (increased R-R interval) that follows the junctional premature complex. This pause or resetting of the sinus node discharge rate is common to all supraventricular ectopic beats.

To review, the three hallmarks of supraventricular premature complexes are (1) the P wave looks different from the normal ones and occurs earlier than expected; (2) the resultant R wave occurs early also but looks similar to the normal R waves; and (3) a compensatory pause occurs before the next P-QRS-T sequence.

The first and seventh QRS complexes are bizarre in appearance and look much different from the others. Note also that these are the same two complexes that have different P-R intervals from the rest (P waves are immediately in front with no P-R *segment* observable). This happens because these are VPCs that have been formed by the firing of injured ventricular cells and subsequent depolarization of the ventricles before the normal P wave activity could be conducted through the normal pathways. Because the pathways involved in the ventricular depolarization were different, the shape of the premature complex is different from that of the normal QRS complex. Note also that they are wider than the normal ones. Because the abnormal impulse is conducted primarily from muscle to muscle, the time required for the impulse to span the ventricle is longer than when the impulse is rapidly conducted through the bundle branches and Purkinje system. Hence, the VPC appears wider (has increased duration) than the normal QRS complexes. They are identified as being ventricular rather than supraventricular because they look so different from the normal QRS complexes.

In summary, this ECG shows an APC and two VPCs. These are common in the first 1 to 5 days following severe trauma and are felt to be associated with bruising of and injury to the atria (APCs) and ventricles (VPCs). Consequently all trauma victims should be carefully screened for the development of dysrhythmias during this period. Recognition of this problem should be brought to the clinician's attention immediately.

Case 7–9 *(Fig. 7–9):*

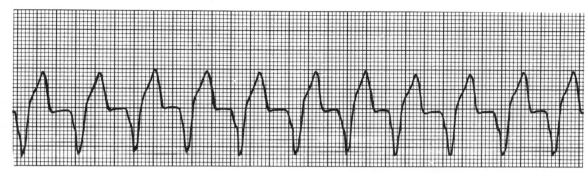

Figure 7–9 ▪ This lead II ECG was recorded from the same 2-year-old mixed breed dog that had been hit by a car in Case 7–8; this ECG was taken 2 hours after the one in Figure 7–8, at a time when the dog had suddenly collapsed. (Paper speed = 50 mm/sec, 1 cm = 1 mv.)

Questions

1. Is the heart rate normal or abnormal?
2. Is the rhythm regular or irregular?
3. Can I identify P waves and QRS complexes?
4. Is there a P wave in front of every QRS complex and a QRS complex following every P wave?
5. Are the p waves and QRS complexes consistently related to each other (P-R intervals all the same)?
6. Do all the P waves look alike and do all the QRS complexes look alike?

Discussion

Question 1. The heart rate calculates out to be approximately 214 beats per minute (3000 divided by 14), which is abnormal.

Question 2. The rhythm appears fairly regular.

Question 3. No P waves can be identified, and no normal-appearing QRS complexes can be seen.

Question 4. Because no P waves are seen, the answer to both questions is "no."

Question 5. There are no P-R intervals because there are no P waves.

Question 6. All of the QRS complexes look alike but they all look bizarre. These are all VPCs. Whenever there are more than three consecutive VPCs, the rhythm is one of ventricular tachycardia. In this case where all of the complexes are VPCs, this is called sustained ventricular tachycardia.

In summary, this ECG represents a typical worsening of the patient's rhythm seen with traumatic myocardial injury and demonstrates the need to monitor such a patient closely. This rhythm can deteriorate rapidly to ventricular fibrillation and death if not recognized and treated immediately. The treatment of choice is lidocaine at a dose of 1 to 2 mg/kg IV push over a 1-minute period followed by a constant-rate infusion of 75 to 100 ug/kg/min adjusted as needed to keep the rhythm normal.

The lidocaine should not contain epinephrine and is usually in a 2 percent solution (strength). This means there are 20 mg of lidocaine per milliliter. Consequently a dose of 2 mg/kg equals 0.1 ml/kg. To approximate the constant-rate infusion of 75 to 100 μg/kg/min, remove 50 ml of fluid from a 1-liter bottle of lactated Ringer's, normal saline, or 5 percent dextrose and water and replace it with 50 ml of 2 percent lidocaine. This provides a concentration of 1 mg/ml or 1000 μg/ml, which would be 0.1 ml/kg/min. Because most standard IV infusion sets provide 20 drops/ml, the drip rate would be 2.0 drops/kg/min. Therefore, a 10-kg dog would get 20 drops/min or 1 drop every 3 sec using a standard IV infusion set. A microdrip IV infusion set provides 60 drops/ml. Therefore, the drip rate for the same 10-kg dog would be 1 drop/sec using the microdrip method. Review these calculations until you understand them thoroughly. In an emergency, there is no time nor margin for errors.

Case 7–10 *(Fig. 7–10A, B):*

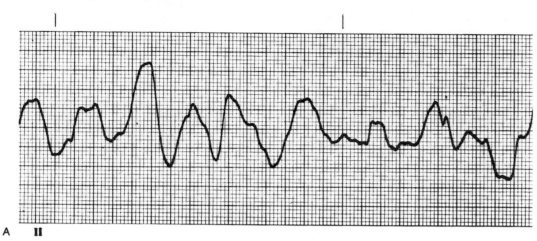

A   **II**

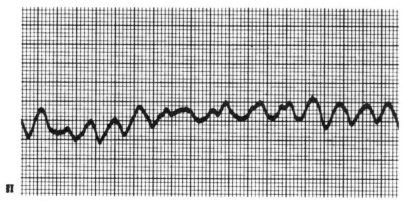

B   **II**

Figure 7–10 ▪ This lead II ECG was recorded from a dog that had just collapsed. (Paper speed = 50 mm/sec, 1 cm = 1 mv.) (From Edwards, NJ: Bolton's Handbook of Canine and Feline Electrocardiography, ed 2. Philadelphia, WB Saunders, 1987, with permission.)

Questions

1. Is the heart rate normal or abnormal?
2. Is the rhythm regular or irregular?
3. Can I identify P waves and QRS complexes?
4. Is there a P wave in front of every QRS complex and a QRS complex following every P wave?
5. Are the P waves and QRS complexes consistently related to each other (P-R intervals all the same)?
6. Do all the P waves look alike and do all the QRS complexes look alike?

Discussion

Question 1. There is no definable pattern to this ECG so the rate cannot be determined.

Question 2. There is marked irregularity in the rhythm, as no two places look the same.

Question 3. Neither P waves or QRS complexes can be identified.

Questions 4, 5, and 6. Because neither P waves or QRS complexes can be identified, all of these must be answered "no."

In summary, you have answered "no" to all six questions. Whenever you have this situation *call for help immediately*, as the patient may be in extreme danger of dying. This ECG represents a chaotic pre-ventricular fibrillatory rhythm that rapidly deteriorated into ventricular fibrillation (see Fig. 7-10B). In this situation you have approximately 2 minutes before death and you *must* learn to recognize this dysrhythmia quickly on visual inspection alone. You *must* immediately institute cardiopulmonary resuscitation and defibrillation for the patient to survive.

SELF-ASSESSMENT

Now that you have reviewed ten ECG cases in a systemic manner, examine each of the following ECG cases and identify the abnormalities. Remember to follow the same steps as you did in cases 7-1 through 7-10. In addition, measure the waveforms for each ECG and, when applicable, estimate the mean electrical axis. When more than one method is available, calculate using all of the methods; familiarize yourself with them. You will find the answers in the appendix (pp. 181-186). Whenever you need to, go back and review the portion of the text dealing with a particular segment of the ECG evaluation. Conclude each problem by formulating what your action plan should be for each case presentation.

Case 7 – 11 *(Fig. 7–11):*

II

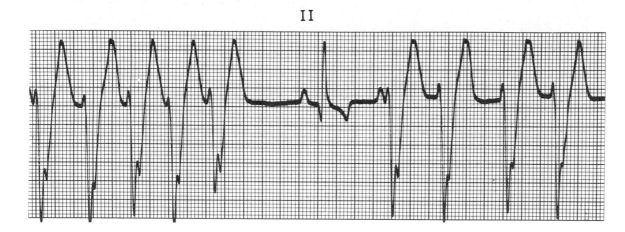

II

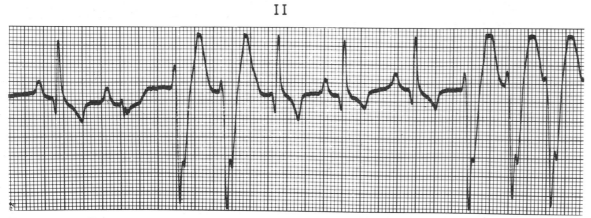

Figure 7 – 11 ▪ These two lead II ECG tracings are continuous and were recorded from a 9-year-old boxer dog with a history of fainting. (Paper speed = 50 mm/sec, 1 cm = 1 mv.)

ECG interpretation for Figure 7–11.

1. Heart rate
2. Rhythm
3. Axis
4. P
   P-R
   QRS
   S-T segment and T wave
   Q-T
5. Miscellaneous criteria
6. Technician action

Case 7 – 12 *(Fig. 7 – 12):*

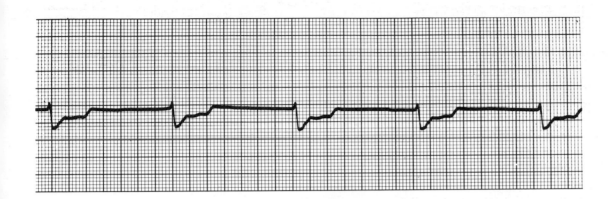

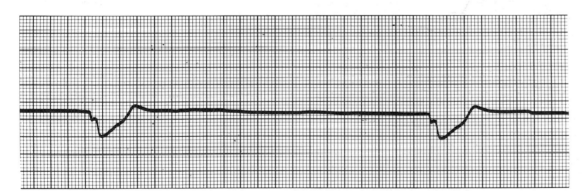

Figure 7 – 12 ▪ These two lead II ECG tracings were recorded from the same dog, a 12-year-old male cocker spaniel, during an anesthetic procedure. The tracings were recorded approximately 4 minutes apart. (Paper speed = 50 mm/sec, 1 cm = 1 mv.)

ECG interpretation for Figure 7–12:

1. Heart rate
2. Rhythm
3. Axis
4. P
   P-R
   QRS
   S-T segment and T wave
   Q-T
5. Miscellaneous criteria
6. Technician action

Case 7 – 13 *(Fig. 7 – 13):*

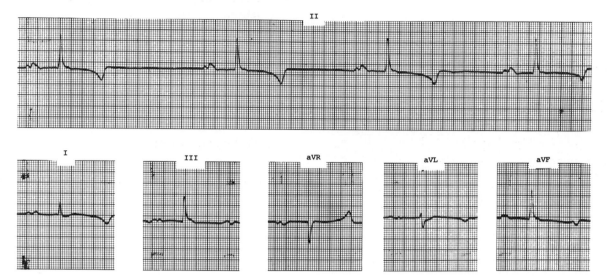

ECG interpretation for Figure 7–13:

1. Heart rate
2. Rhythm
3. Axis
4. P
   P-R
   QRS
   S-T segment and T wave
   Q-T
5. Miscellaneous criteria
6. Technician action

Figure 7 – 13 ▪ This ECG was recorded from an Arabian yearling with a loud murmur. (Paper speed = 50 mm/ sec, 1 cm = 1 mv.)

Case 7 – 14 *(Fig. 7 – 14):*

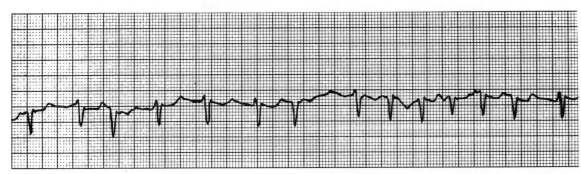

Figure 7 – 14 ▪ This lead II ECG was recorded from a 13-year-old DSH cat with systemic hypertension. (Paper speed = 50 mm/sec, 1 cm = 1 mv.)

ECG interpretation for Figure 7 – 14:

1. Heart rate
2. Rhythm
3. Axis
4. P
   P-R
   QRS
   S-T segment and T wave
   Q-T
5. Miscellaneous criteria
6. Technician action

Case 7 – 15 *(Fig. 7 – 15):*

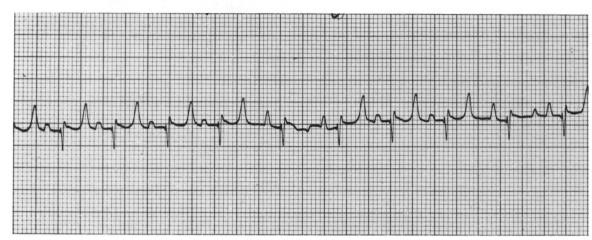

Figure 7 – 15 ▪ This lead II ECG was recorded from a 3-day-old Holstein calf with a large ventricular septal defect. (Paper speed = 25 mm/sec, 1 cm = 1 mv.)

ECG interpretation for Figure 7–15:

1. Heart rate
2. Rhythm
3. Axis
4. P
   P-R
   QRS
   S-T segment and T wave
   Q-T
5. Miscellaneous criteria
6. Technician action

Case 7 – 16 *(Fig. 7 – 16):*

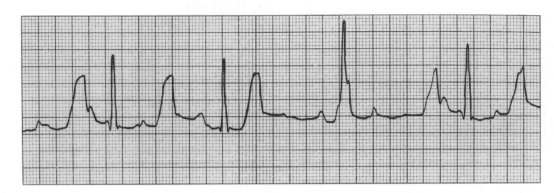

ECG interpretation for Figure 7–16:

1. Heart rate
2. Rhythm
3. Axis
4. P
   P-R
   QRS
   S-T segment and T wave
   Q-T
5. Miscellaneous criteria
6. Technician action

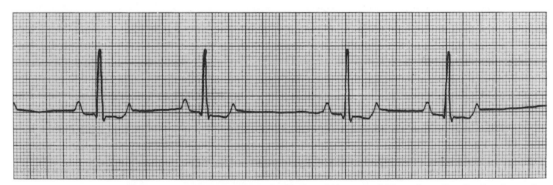

Figure 7 – 16 ▪ The top lead II ECG tracing was recorded from a 1½-year-old female rottweiler having seizures. The lower lead II ECG tracing is from the same dog 24 hours later. (Paper speed = 50 mm/sec, 1 cm = 1 mv.)

Case 7 – 17 *(Fig. 7–17):*

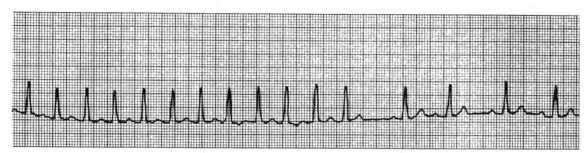

Figure 7 – 17 ▪ This lead II ECG tracing was recorded from a 3-year-old male boxer dog with syncope (fainting episodes). (Paper speed = 50 mm/sec, 1 cm = 1 mv.)

ECG interpretation for Figure 7–17:

1. Heart rate
2. Rhythm
3. Axis
4. P
   P-R
   QRS
   S-T segment and T wave
   Q-T
5. Miscellaneous criteria
6. Technician action

Case 7 – 18 *(Fig. 7 – 18):*

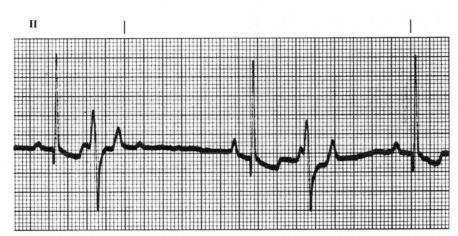

Figure 7 – 18 ▪ This lead II ECG was recorded from a dog undergoing anesthesia induction by intravenous thiamyl sodium injection. (Paper speed = 50 mm/sec, 1 cm = 1 mv.) (From Edwards, NJ: Bolton's Handbook of Canine and Feline Electrocardiography, ed 2. Philadelphia, WB Saunders, 1987, with permission.)

ECG interpretation for Figure 7 – 18:

1. Heart rate
2. Rhythm
3. Axis
4. P
   P-R
   QRS
   S-T segment and T wave
   Q-T
5. Miscellaneous criteria
6. Technician action

Case 7 – 19 *(Fig. 7 – 19):*

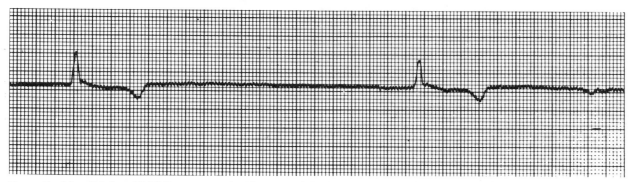

Figure 7 – 19 ▪ This lead II ECG was recorded from a cat that was semicomatose with a urethral obstruction. (Paper speed = 50 mm/sec, 1 cm = 1 mv.) (From Edwards, NJ: Bolton's Handbook of Canine and Feline Electrocardiography, ed 2. Philadelphia, WB Saunders, 1987, with permission.)

ECG Interpretation for Figure 7 – 19:

1. Heart rate
2. Rhythm
3. Axis
4. P
   P-R
   QRS
   S-T segment and T wave
   Q-T
5. Miscellaneous criteria
6. Technician action

Case 7–20 *(Fig. 7–20):*

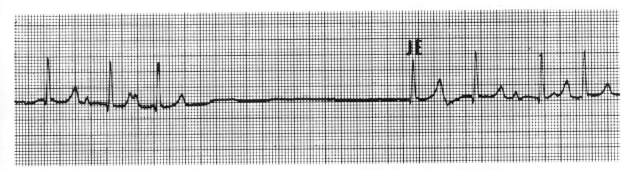

Figure 7–20 ▪ Lead II ECG was recorded from a 13-year-old female cocker spaniel with a history of syncope. (Paper speed = 50 mm/sec, 1 cm = 1 mv.) (From Edwards, NJ: Bolton's Handbook of Canine and Feline Electrocardiography, ed 2. Philadelphia, WB Saunders, 1987, with permission.)

ECG interpretation for Figure 7–20:

1. Heart rate
2. Rhythm
3. Axis
4. P
   P-R
   QRS
   S-T segment and T wave
   Q-T
5. Miscellaneous criteria
6. Technician action

The remainder of this chapter will consist of examples of typical ECG recordings in different species. Each will be identified with an ECG diagnosis. Apply the principles you have learned in the preceding chapters and in the first portion of this one to formulate a *technician action* for each example. Remember, it is more important to recognize an ECG as being abnormal and in need of immediate attention by a veterinary clinician than it is to be able to make a complete ECG diagnosis for detailed discussion at the next staff meeting. It is important to realize that, as some of these ECG patterns will be displayed moving across a monitor screen, prompt recognition of changes in the baseline ECG may well save the patient's life. Here again, recognizing that there is a change and how serious it may be is more important than being able to lecture profusely on the specific ECG diagnosis. In general, pay more attention to the rhythm and the uniformity of the P-QRS-T sequence than to the measurement of waveforms, segments, and intervals. Remember these few rules and electrocardiography will be fun.

Rule 1:   Don't panic!

Rule 2:   The first pulse to take in an emergency is your own.

Rule 3:   The more "no" answers you get to the six basic questions about the P-QRS-T sequence, the faster you should get help.

Numerous texts in the veterinary and human medical literature have been published on electrocardiography. Use them to expand your knowledge and understanding once you have mastered the basics presented in this text. With knowledge and experience will come wisdom and confidence. Remember the words of Solomon: "Get all the knowledge you can and you will succeed; without it, you will fail."

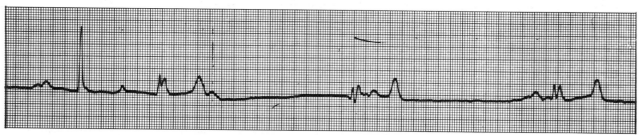

Figure 7–21 ▪ This lead II ECG was recorded from a horse. (Paper speed = 50 mm/sec, 1 cm = 1 mv.) ECG diagnosis: Three VPCs are seen following a normal P-QRS-T sequence.

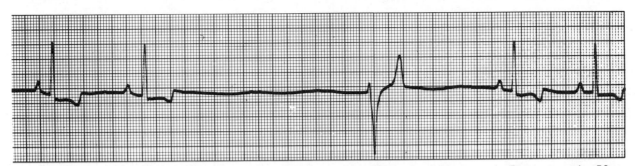

Figure 7–22 ▪ This lead II ECG was recorded from a dog with fainting spells (syncope). (Paper speed = 50 mm/sec, 1 cm = 1 mv.) ECG diagnosis: Ventricular escape beat occurring during a period of sinus arrest. S-T segment depression is also evident in the normal P-QRS-T sequence.

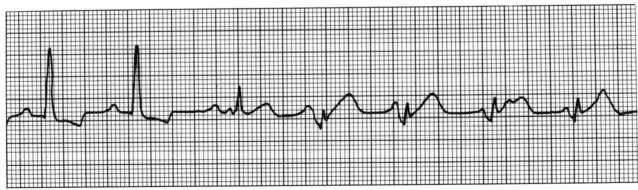

Figure 7–23 ▪ This lead II ECG was recorded from a dog. (Paper speed = 50 mm/sec, 1 cm = 1 mv.) ECG diagnosis: Two normal P-QRS-T sequences, followed by a "ventricular fusion beat" and 4 VPCs.

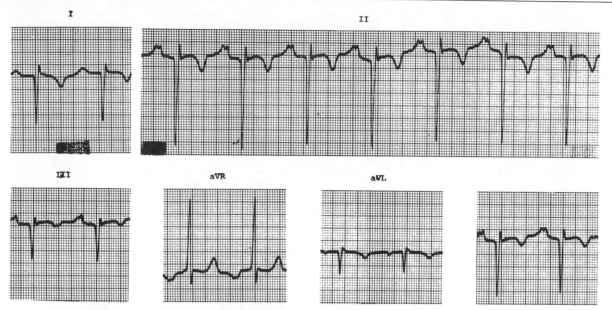

Figure 7–24 ■ This ECG was recorded from a 3-week-old standardbred foal with cyanosis. (Paper speed = 25 mm/sec, 1 cm = 1 mv.) ECG diagnosis: P mitrale. Marked deviation of initial depolarization forces to the right.

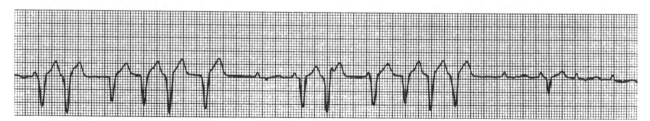

Figure 7–25 ■ This lead II ECG was recorded from a 12-year-old DSH Cat. (Paper speed = 50 mm/sec, 1 cm = 1 mv.) ECG diagnosis: Ventricular tachycardia. The P waves are easily seen, but the QRS is barely visible in the four normal P-QRS-T sequences.

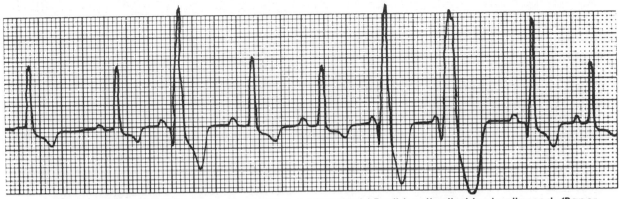

Figure 7–26 ■ This lead II ECG was recorded from a 13-year-old English setter that had collapsed. (Paper speed = 50 mm/sec, 1 cm = 1 mv.) ECG diagnosis: The third and eighth complexes are fusion beats. Note the P wave in front of each. The sixth and seventh complexes are VPCs.

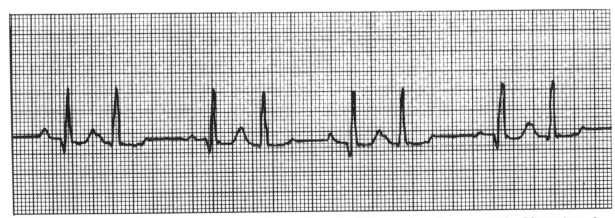

Figure 7–27 ■ This lead II ECG was recorded from a 5-month-old boxer dog. (Paper speed = 50 mm/sec, 1 cm = 1 mv.) ECG diagosis: Atrial bigeminy. Every other complex beginning with the second one is an APC.

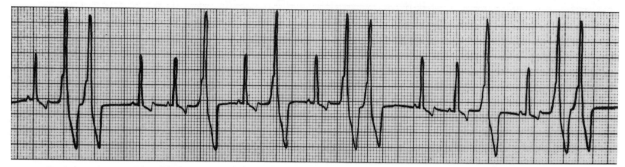

Figure 7 – 28 ▪ This lead II ECG was recorded from a 13-year-old boxer dog that was experiencing syncope. (Paper speed = 25 mm/sec, 1 cm = 1 mv.) ECG diagnosis: Multiple VPCs occurring in singles and pairs.

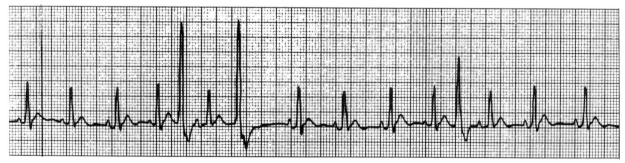

Figure 7 – 29 ▪ This lead II ECG was recorded from a 6-year-old ferret with dilative cardiomyopathy. (Paper speed = 50 mm/sec, 1 cm = 1 mv.) ECG diagnosis: Multiform VPCs.

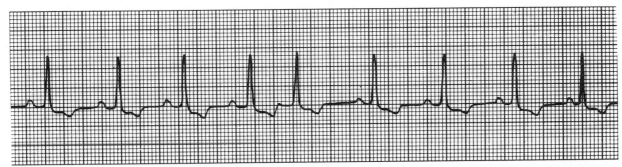

Figure 7–30 ▪ This lead II ECG was recorded from an aged dog. (Paper speed = 50 mm/sec, 1 cm = 1 mv.) ECG diagnosis: An APC is seen (fifth complex from the left).

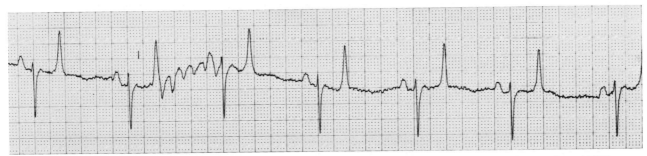

Figure 7–31 ▪ This base-apex ECG was recorded from a cow. (Paper speed = 25 mm/sec, 1 cm = 1 mv.) ECG diagnosis: Muscular twitching artifact.

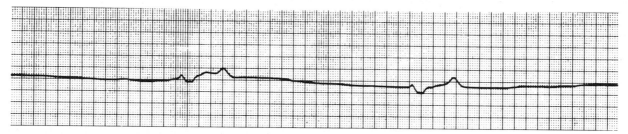

Figure 7–32 ▪ This lead II ECG was recorded from a cat. (Paper speed = 50 mm/sec, 1 cm = 1 mv.) ECG diagnosis: Electromechanical dissociation (ventricular arrest). (From Edwards, NJ: Bolton's Handbook of Canine and Feline Electrocardiography, ed 2. Philadelphia, WB Saunders, 1987, with permission.)

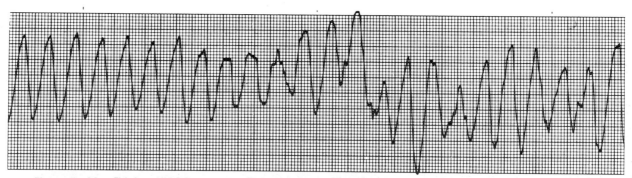

Figure 7–33 ▪ This lead II ECG was recorded from a cat. (Paper speed = 50 mm/sec, 1 cm = 1 mv.) ECG diagnosis: Bizarre ventricular tachycardia. This is a prefibrillation rhythm. (From Edwards, NJ: Bolton's Handbook of Canine and Feline Electrocardiography, ed 2. Philadelphia, WB Saunders, 1987, with permission.)

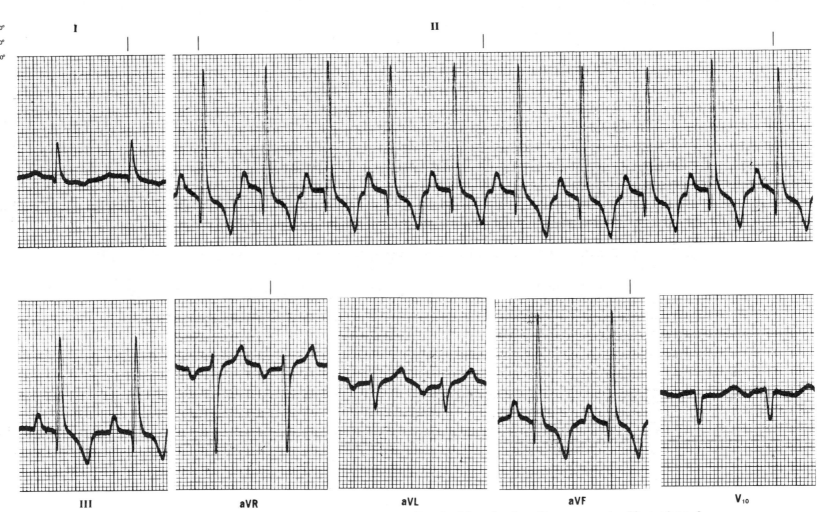

Figure 7–34 ▪ This ECG was recorded from an aged Standard Poodle dog. (Paper speed = 50 mm/sec, 1 cm = 1 mv.) ECG diagnosis: Supraventricular tachycardia. (From Edwards, NJ: Bolton's Handbook of Canine and Feline Electrocardiography, ed 2. Philadelphia, WB Saunders, 1987, with permission.)

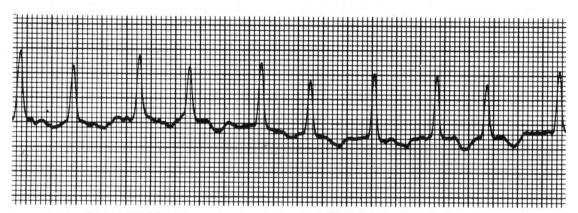

Figure 7 – 35 ▪ This lead II ECG was recorded from a 5-year-old DSH cat. (Paper speed = 50 mm/sec, 1 cm = 1 mv.) ECG diagnosis: Atrial fibrillation. (From Edwards, NJ: Bolton's Handbook of Canine and Feline Electrocardiography, ed 2. Philadelphia, WB Saunders, 1987, with permission.)

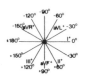

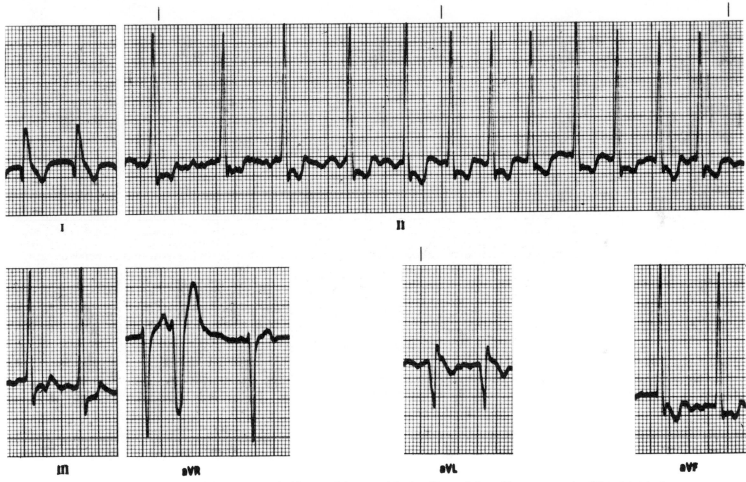

I   II

III   aVR   aVL   aVF

Figure 7–36 ▪ This ECG was recorded from a 14-year-old mixed breed dog. (Paper speed = 50 mm/sec, 1 cm = 1 mv.) ECG diagnosis: Atrial fibrillation with one VPC seen in lead aVR. (From Edwards, NJ: Bolton's Handbook of Canine and Feline Electrocardiography, ed 2. Philadelphia, WB Saunders, 1987, with permission.)

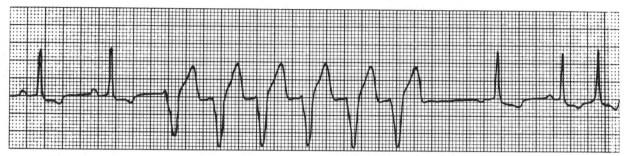

Figure 7–37 ▪ This lead II ECG was recorded on a dog. (Paper speed = 50 mm/sec, 1 cm = 1 mv.) ECG diagnosis: Ventricular tachycardia. Two junctional beats are seen: one is a junctional escape complex seen after the burst of ventricular tachycardia, and one is a premature junctional complex (last complex on right).

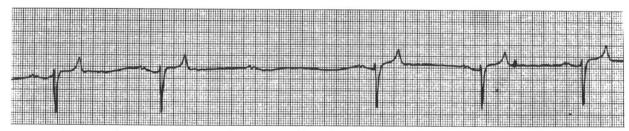

Figure 7–38 ▪ This base-apex lead was recorded from a miniature horse. (Paper speed = 25 mm/sec, 1 cm = 1 mv.) ECG diagnosis: Second-degree A-V block.

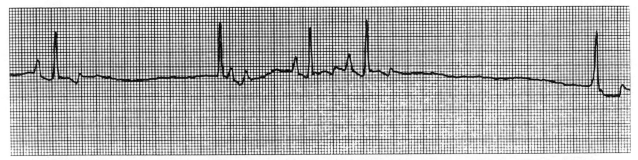

Figure 7–39 ▪ This lead II ECG was recorded from a 13-year-old female cocker spaniel dog. (Paper speed = 50 mm/sec, 1 cm = 1 mv.) ECG diagnosis: Sick sinus syndrome (periods of sinus arrest followed by escape beats). Note the P wave in the S-T segment of the first escape beat.

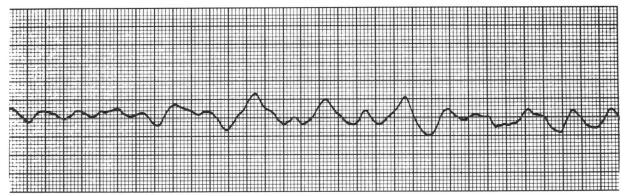

Figure 7–40 ▪ This lead II ECG was recorded from a dog. (Paper speed = 50 mm/sec, 1 cm = 1 mv.) ECG Diagnosis: Ventricular Fibrillation.

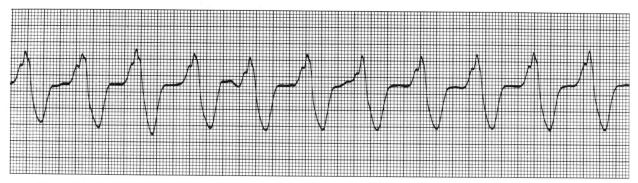

Figure 7–41 ▪ This lead II ECG was recorded from a dog. (Paper speed = 50 mm/sec, 1 cm = 1 mv.) ECG diagnosis: Ventricular tachycardia.

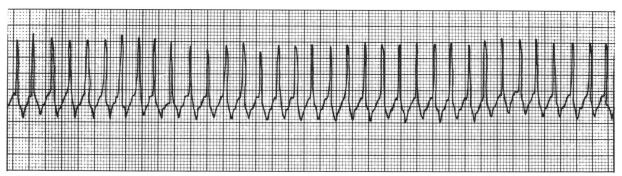

Figure 7–42 ▪ This lead II ECG was recorded from a ferret. (Paper speed = 50 mm/sec, 1 cm = 1 mv.) ECG diagnosis: Supraventricular tachycardia.

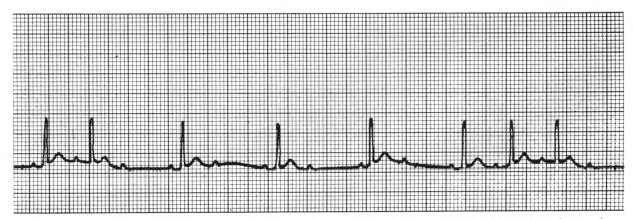

Figure 7–43 ▪ This lead II ECG was recorded from a 2-year-old ferret. (Paper speed = 50 mm/sec, 1 cm = 1 mv.) ECG diagnosis: Second-degree A-V block.

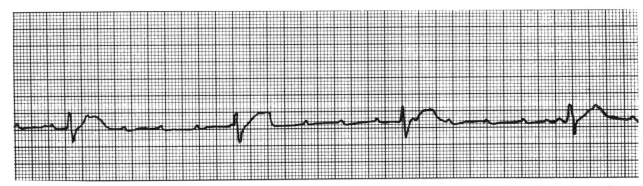

Figure 7–44 ▪ This lead II ECG was recorded from a 3-year-old ferret. (Paper speed = 50 mm/sec, 1 cm = 1 mv.) ECG diagnosis: Third-degree A-V block.

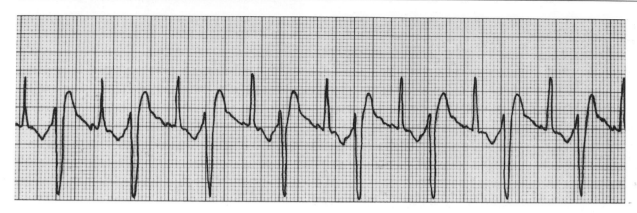

Figure 7-45 ▪ This lead II ECG was recorded from a 5 year old ferret. (Paper speed = 50 mm/sec, 1 cm = 1 mv.) ECG diagnosis: Ventricular bigeminy.

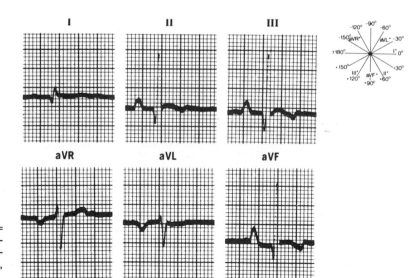

Figure 7-46 ▪ Normal canine ECG. (Paper speed = 50 mm/sec, 1 cm = 1 mv.) (From Edwards, NJ: Bolton's Handbook of Canine and Feline Electrocardiography, ed 2. Philadelphia, WB Saunders, 1987, with permission.)

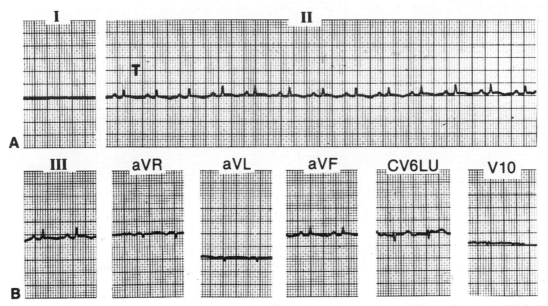

Figure 7–47 ▪ Normal feline ECG. (Paper speed = 50 mm/sec, 1 cm = 1 mv.) (From Edwards, NJ: Bolton's Handbook of Canine and Feline Electrocardiography, ed 2. Philadelphia, WB Saunders, 1987, with permission.)

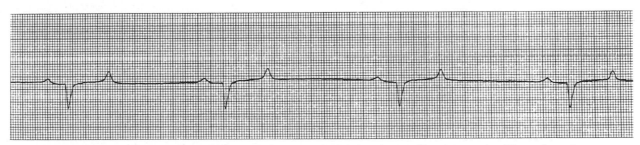

Figure 7–48 ▪ Base-apex lead recorded from a normal miniature horse. (Paper speed = 50 mm/sec, 1 cm = 1 mv.)

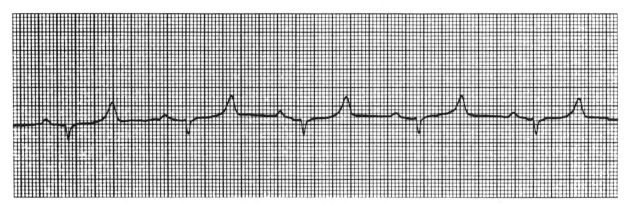

Figure 7–49 ▪ Base-apex ECG recorded from a normal sheep. (Paper speed = 50 mm/sec, 1 cm = 1 mv.)

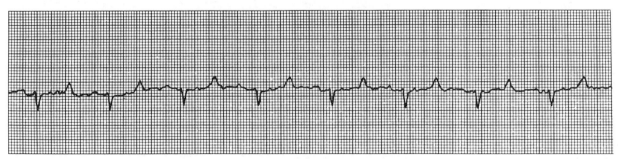

Figure 7–50 ▪ Base-apex ECG recorded from a normal goat. (Paper speed = 50 mm/sec, 1 cm = 1 mv.)

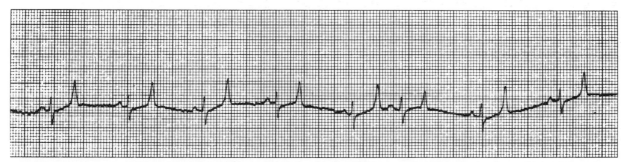

Figure 7–51 ▪ Base-apex ECG recorded from a normal llama. (Paper speed = 25 mm/sec, 1 cm = 1 mv.)

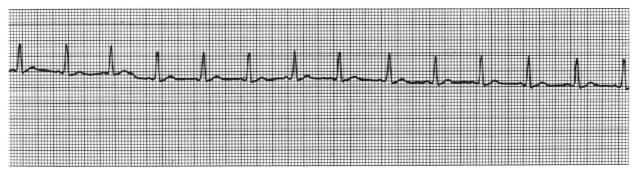

Figure 7–52 ▪ Lead II ECG recorded from a normal ferret. (Paper speed = 50 mm/sec, 1 cm = 1 mv.)

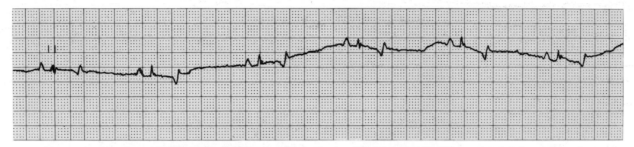

Figure 7–53 ▪ Lead II ECG recorded from a normal cow. (Paper speed = 25 mm/sec, 1 cm = 1 mv.)

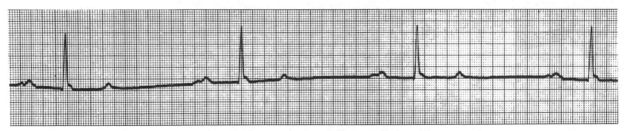

Figure 7–54 ▪ Lead II ECG recorded from a normal horse. (Paper speed = 50 mm/sec, 1 cm = 1 mv.).

Complete (Third-Degree) Heart Block The most severe form of heart block, in which atrial impulses are blocked at the A-V node. On the ECG the atria beat at their own rate and the ventricles beat at their own rate, which is almost always slower than the atrial rate. There is no relationship between P waves and QRS complexes.

APC Atrial premature complex formed by the electrical discharge of an atrial site outside the S-A node. The P wave may appear different from the regular P wave. It is conducted through normal pathways in the ventricle so the QRS, although occurring early (premature), looks similar to the normal QRS complex. This premature complex is usually followed by a compensatory pause before the next sinus node discharge.

VPC (PVC) (VPD) Ventricular premature complex; this is a premature depolarization arising from an ectopic site below the A-V node. Usually the QRS formed by a VPC is bizarre in shape and prolonged in duration.

Second-Degree A-V Block Some atrial impulses (P waves) are conducted through the A-V node and depolarize the ventricles; others are blocked at the A-V node and do not cause depolarization of the ventricles. There are two types of second-degree A-V block. Type I (Mobitz type I) or Wenckebach A-V block is seen as a progressive lengthening of the P-R interval until a P wave eventually is unable to be conducted to the ventricle (because it is blocked). Type II (Mobitz type II) is seen as periodic blocking of P-wave transmission through the A-V node without a change in the P-R interval of those P waves that are not blocked.

Atrial Fibrillation No P waves are seen on the ECG and the baseline is usually irregular owing to many (more than five) chaotic wavefronts (wavelets) traveling randomly in the atrial myocardium. The ventricular depolarization rate is usually irregular and rapid as these wavelets (f waves) bombard the A-V node.

Ventricular Tachycardia A series of four or more VPCs in succession.

Right Bundle Branch Block Blockage of impulse conduction through the right branch of the bundle of His, resulting in a delay in depolarization of the right ventricle. This causes prolongation (widening) of the terminal forces of the QRS complex, which results in wide jagged or notched S waves.

Ventricular Fibrillation Disorganized electrical activity in the ventricles characterized on the ECG as bizarre baseline undulations. No P waves or QRS complexes are seen. No mechanical pumping (beating) of the heart is present.

Electromechanical Dissociation Wide bizarre QRS complexes occurring at a very slow rate are seen on the ECG, but the electrical stimulus causes no mechanical contraction of the heart.

Paroxysmal Atrial Tachycardia (PAT) Burst of four or more consecutive APCs that start and end abruptly with a return to normal S-A node depolarization.

Ventricular Bigeminy A condition in which every other beat is a VPC, alternating between normal and abnormal ventricular depolarization.

Hyperkalemia Elevated serum or plasma levels of potassium.

Sick Sinus Syndrome A disease of the S-A node and the atria characterized by sinus bradycardia, sinus arrest, APCs, or supraventricular tachycardia occurring in the same ECG.

Fusion Beat A QRS complex that is formed as the normal impulse and an ectopic ventricular impulse simultaneously cause ventricular depolarization. it is seen on the ECG as a P wave followed by a QRS complex whose shape is midway between that of the normal QRS complex and that of the VPC.

Mobitz Type I A-V Block See Second-Degree A-V Block.

Wenckebach A-V Block This is the same as Mobitz type I A-V block; see Second Degree A-V Block.

Capture Beat The first normal P-QRS-T sequence following a string of VPCs.

Ventricular Escape Beat An ectopic impulse originating from the ventricles following a long pause in the rhythm owing to failure of S-A node depolarization or failure of conduction to the ventricles. Although on the ECG these will appear as VPCs, they are not really "premature" but rather occur *after* a pause in the rhythm.

Junctional Escape Beat An ectopic impulse originating from the junctional tissue around the A-V node following a long pause in the rhythm. The QRS and T waves are usually normal in appearance. The P

wave is usually negative or is undetectable.

Constant-Rate Infusion The IV administration of drugs and/or fluids at a consistent volume or strength throughout a given period of time.

Vagal Maneuver The use of ocular pressure or carotid sinus massage to correct a dysrhythmia through an increase in vagal tone (stimulation).

Tachycardia A rapid heart rate above normal for the species being examined.

Bradycardia A slow heart rate below normal for the species being examined.

Artificial Pacemaker Implantation The act of placing a battery-powered electronic device connected by a pacing electrode wire to the heart that generates a spike of current that will depolarize the ventricles, consequently sustaining an effective cardiac rhythm. These units consist of a battery (pacemaker) that is surgically placed under the skin or in the abdomen and a lead wire system that is either passed through the jugular vein into the heart or connected surgically directly to the exterior of the ventricular wall (epicardium).

References

Conover, MB: Understanding Electrocardiography, Arrhythmias and the 12-lead ECG, ed 5. St Louis, CV Mosby, 1988.

Edwards, NJ: Bolton's Handbook of Canine and Feline Electrocardiography, ed 2. Philadelphia, WB Saunders, 1987.

Tilley, LP: Essentials of Canine and Feline Electrocardiography. Philadelphia, Lea and Febiger, 1985.

Tilley, LP, Smith, FWK, and Miller, MS: Cardiology Pocket Reference. Denver, American Animal Hospital Association, 1990.

Appendix

ANSWERS TO CASE STUDIES CHAPTER 5

CASE 5-1

1. No, too many artifacts are present.

2. (a) Wandering of the baseline, (b) patient movement, (c) inability to clearly see the R wave deflection.

3. (a) and (b) Provide improved restraint by calming the patient, holding the patient more firmly, repositioning the leads, and/or placing the patient in a more comfortable position. (c) Increase the stylus heat and clean the stylus debris, if necessary.

CASE 5-2

1. (a) 60-cycle electrical interference, (b) baseline movement associated with respiratory movement, (c) abrupt gross patient movement resulting in two large negative (downward) deflections in the middle of the tracing. (These were caused by leg jerking by the patient.)

2. Yes, artifacts are present. There are unexplained positive (upward) deflections that resemble P waves, occurring regularly throughout this ECG. One occurs immediately before the first and second QRS complexes. They are also seen between QRS complexes and immediately following the last QRS complex on the right. These are muscular twitch artifacts. If you were in doubt when you observed these during the recording, they could be identified by manually pressing the lead marker button to coincide with observed patient movement.

CASE 5-3

1. Muscular trembling artifacts are seen. This patient was nervous and would alternately tremble and relax. Note that the very beginning and very end of the recording is reasonably free of artifacts during periods of relaxation. The muscular trembling begins during the S-T segment of the second complex of the top tracing and continues until the last two complexes of the lower tracing.

2. Corrections might be accomplished by calming the patient, or applying comforting firm pressure over the body, being careful not to touch the electrodes. Note the difference in appearance of this baseline compared with the 60-cycle electrical interference in Figure 5-6.

CASE 5-4

1. Muscular trembling artifact and baseline movement artifact caused by patient movement. Note the lower ECG tracing was recorded on the same patient following tranquilization. Now all wave forms and intervals can be seen clearly.

CASE 5-5

1. This is a baseline movement artifact due to panting. Note the bizarre rapid stylus movement that makes it impossible to read this ECG.

2. a. Place a roll of paper towels between the patient's legs.
   b. Close the patient's mouth.
   c. Calm and comfort the patient.

d. Apply direct thoracic and leg restraints to minimize body movement during panting.

e. Tranquilize the patient, if necessary.

In this case, a paper towel roll was placed between the patient's forelegs and rear legs to minimize electrode movement during panting.

Note the lower tracing has some remaining wave-like undulations in the baseline. However, marked improvement has resulted from this single technique.

CASE 5–6

1. 60-cycle electrical interference.
2. Refer to the 14 steps outlined in the section of the text that discusses 60-cycle electrical interference.

CHAPTER 6: ECG INTERPRETATIONS

ECG interpretation for Figure 6–69:

1. Heart rate = 176 (R-R interval is 17 boxes, divided into 3000)
2. Rhythm = normal sinus rhythm (NSR)
3. Axis = +90°
4. Measure and multiply:
   P = 0.04 sec (2 boxes by 0.3 mv (3 boxes)
   P-R = 0.10 sec (5 boxes)
   QRS = 0.05 sec (2½ boxes) by 1.9 mv (19 boxes)

S-T segment and T wave = normal
Q-T = 0.16 sec (8 boxes)
5. Miscellaneous criteria: none
6. Electrocardiographic diagnosis: normal.

ECG interpretation for Figure 6–70:

1. Heart rate = 111 to 120 (shortest R-R is 25 boxes, longest is 27 boxes)
2. Rhythm = sinus arrhythmia (R-R varies slightly)
3. Axis = +150° (if lead II is used as isoelectric), +180° (if lead aVF is used as isoelectric). It may be averaged at +165°.
4. Measure and multiply:
   P = 0.04 sec (2 boxes by 0.2 mv (2 boxes)
   P-R = 0.13 to 0.14 sec
   QRS = 0.05 sec (2½ boxes) by 0.5 mv (5 boxes)
   S-T segment and T wave = normal
   Q-T = 0.18 sec (9 boxes)
5. Miscellaneous criteria: S_1, S_2, S_3 pattern (S waves present in leads I, II, and III); deep S wave in lead CV_6LU (S wave deeper than 0.7 mv)
6. Electrocardiographic diagnosis: right axis deviation; S_1, S_2, S_3 pattern (right ventricular enlargement); deep S wave in lead CCV_6LU

ECG interpretation for Figure 6–71:

1. Heart rate = 230 (R-R is 13 boxes)
2. Rhythm = NSR
3. Axis = +90°

4. Measure and multiply:
   P = 0.04 sec (2 boxes) × 0.15 mv (1½ boxes)
   P-R = 0.08 (4 boxes)
   QRS = 0.04 sec (2 boxes) × 0.4 mv (4 boxes)
   S-T segment and T wave = normal
   Q-T = 0.16 sec (8 boxes) (best seen in CV_6LU)
5. Miscellaneous criteria: none
6. Electrocardiographic diagnosis: normal

ECG interpretation for Figure 6–72:

1. Heart rate = 230 (R-R is 13 boxes)
2. Rhythm = normal sinus rhythm
3. Axis = +100°
4. Measure and multiply:
   P = 0.04 sec (2 boxes) × 0.15 mv (1½ boxes)
   P-R = 0.06 (3 boxes)
   QRS = 0.04 sec (2 boxes) × 1.3 mv (13 boxes)
   S-T segment and T wave = normal
   Q-T = 0.14 sec (7 boxes) (as determined by measuring from Q to the return to baseline preceding the next P wave)
5. Miscellaneous criteria: none
6. Electrocardiographic diagnosis: left ventricular enlargement

ECG interpretation for Figure 6–73:

1. Heart rate = 231 (R-R interval = 13 boxes divided into 3000)
2. Rhythm = NSR
3. Axis = impossible to determine because

only one lead is shown. All of the methods described require at least two leads in the frontal plane to determine the mean electrical axis.

4. Measure and multiply:
   P = 0.02 sec (1 box) × 0.1 mv (1 box)
   P-R = 0.05 sec (2½ boxes)
   QRS = 0.04 sec (2 boxes) × 1.7 mv (17 boxes)
   S-T segment = normal (approximately 0.02 sec duration [1 box])
   T wave = 0.06 sec (3 boxes) × 0.15 mv (1½ boxes)
   Q-T = 0.13 sec (6½ boxes)
5. Miscellaneous criteria: none
6. Electrocardiographic diagnosis: normal lead II for the ferret

ECG interpretation for Figure 6–74:

1. Heart rate = 38 when lead II is used, 40 when the base-apex lead is used
2. Rhythm = NSR
3. Axis = approximately +60° (aVL is isoelectric, lead II is perpendicular to aVL and lead II is positive)
4. Measure and multiply:
   P = 0.16 sec (8 boxes)
   P-R = 0.44 sec (22 boxes)
   QRS = 0.08 sec (4 boxes)
   S-T segment = 0.28 sec (14 boxes)
   T wave = 0.14 sec (7 boxes)
   Q-T = 0.50 sec (25 boxes)
5. Miscellaneous criteria: amplitudes were not measured because they are not dependable indicator of heart size in the horse
6. Electrocardiographic diagnosis: normal

ECG interpretation for Figure 6–75:

1. Heart rate = 42 to 45 beats per minute
2. Rhythm = sinus arrhythmia
3. Axis = not calculated in the frontal plane for the cow
4. Measure and multiply:
   P = 0.08 sec × 0.2 mv
   P-R = 0.18 sec
   QRS = 0.08 sec × 0.4 mv
   S-T segment and T wave = biphasic T wave
   Q-T = 0.44 sec
5. Miscellaneous criteria: note how much clearer the waveforms appear in the base-apex lead
6. Electrocardiographic diagnosis: Normal ECG for the cow

Fine muscular tremor artifacts are present throughout the recording, resulting in a slightly irregular baseline.

CHAPTER 7: ECG INTERPRETATIONS

CASE 7–11

1. Heart rate: The sinus rate is approximately 160 beats/min, but the actual heart rate varies between 160 and nearly 300 beats/min, as the rhythm is not always a sinus rhythm.
2. Rhythm: The rhythm is irregular, owing to the presence of many bizarre QRS complexes that have no P waves associated with them.

3. Axis: The axis cannot be calculated, as only lead II is present.
4. P = 0.04 sec × 0.3 mv
   P-R = 0.10 sec
   QRS = 0.07 sec × 1.6 mv (qR pattern)
   S-T segment and T wave = ST segment slurring present, T wave somewhat variable
   Q-T = 0.18 sec
5. Miscellaneous criteria: The major problem in this ECG strip is the presence of many ventricular premature complexes (VPCs) that markedly affect the rhythm. Note the second complex from the left on the lower ECG. This is a fusion beat formed by simultaneous depolarization of the ventricle by the normal sinus impulse (note the normal P wave) and the abnormal ectopic focus (VPC). Notice how the shape of the QRS is small and jagged and appears somewhere between the shape of the normal QRS and the VPC.
6. Technician action: This is ventricular tachycardia, a serious dysrhythmia; the clinician should be notified immediately. Intravenous (IV) lidocaine, first as a bolus and then as a constant-rate infusion, should be prepared for administration.

CASE 7–12

1. Heart rate: 100 beats/min in the top strip; 40 beats/min in the lower strip.
2. Rhythm: Although this rhythm is regular, no P waves can be seen and the QRS shape and width appear bizarre and excessively wide.

3. Axis: The axis cannot be calculated, as only lead II is present.

4. P = none seen

P-R = cannot calculate

QRS = Top, 0.10 sec × −0.6 mv; lower, unable to measure, S-T segment and T wave = S-T segment is depressed and unclear as to where it stops because of the lack of a clear T wave in both the upper and lower tracings.

Q-T = Estimated at 0.24 sec on the top tracing and 0.32 sec on the lower tracing.

5. Miscellaneous criteria: The major problem in the top ECG tracing is the lack of any atrial activity (P waves) and slow, bizarre, wide yet regular ventricular activity (QRS complex). This is sinoventricular rhythm (no atrial activity is seen), which is always a very serious sign of impending disaster. It is most often seen with severe hyperkalemia or severe myocardial toxicity (in this case, from the anesthesia). The lower tracing represents a ventricular escape rhythm. No mechanical contraction is occurring at this time and therefore electromechanical dissociation is said to be present.

6. Technician action: When the top tracing was recorded, immediate cessation of anesthesia and initiation of emergency support including IV fluids, drugs for shock, and oxygen should have been instituted. At the time of the lower tracing, the patient was in cardiopulmonary arrest and resuscitation was in progress. This patient died within a few minutes. Prompt recognition of impending tragedy when the top tracing was recorded might have saved the patient's life.

CASE 7 – 13

1. Heart rate: 38 to 42 beats/min

2. Rhythm: sinus arrhythmia

3. Axis: Usually the mean electrical axis is not calculated in the frontal plane for the horse. However, it appears to be approximately +60° if an axis were calculated.

4. P = 0.12 sec × 0.2 mv, notched

P-R = 0.28 sec

QRS = 0.06 sec; remember, the amplitudes are not meaningful in the horse

S-T segment and T wave = The S-T segment appears isoelectric, concluding in a T wave that lasts approximately 0.12 sec

Q-T = 0.48 sec

5. Miscellaneous criteria: There is a normal rate, rhythm, shape, and sequence of waveforms, consistently related to each other.

6. Technician action: No action is required with respect to the ECG, as it appears normal for the horse. Did you recognize it immediately as a horse? Remember that the notched P waves are normal for the horse. The murmur in this yearling horse was due to an atrial septal defect. There were no symptoms present.

CASE 7 – 14

1. Heart rate: Approximately 240 beats/min

2. Rhythm: Irregular, without any pattern

3. Axis: Unable to calculate, as only lead II is seen

4. P = None seen

P-R = unable to calculate because no P wave present

QRS = 0.05 sec × −0.7 mv (QS or rS pattern)

S-T segment and T wave = T waves appear variable

Q-T = Estimate at 0.16 sec

5. Miscellaneous criteria: The important observation in this ECG is a very rapid, irregular rhythm, without evidence of P waves. Note also there are slight variations in the shape of the QRS complex. These are hallmarks of atrial fibrillation. Note also the QRS complex is negative in this strip. Normally the lead II QRS is positive in the cat. Although you cannot tell from this lead alone, this cat had severe left ventricular hypertrophy and also had a left anterior fascicular block, which is responsible for the rS pattern to the QRS complex. Review Figure 6–55.

6. Technician action: The technician should recognize an irregular rapid heart rate and should simultaneously auscultate the heart and palpate the femoral pulse. Almost always more heartbeats are heard than femoral pulses are felt (pulse deficits). Atrial fibrillation is a significant dysrhythmia in the cat and is almost always associated with severe cardiac enlargement or hypertrophy. Pulmonary edema and dyspnea are frequently present and the patients do not tolerate excessive stress and handling. Procedures such as

drawing blood, x-ray examinations, blood pressure recording, and so on should be carried out slowly and carefully with a minimum amount of stress and restraint.

CASE 7-15

1. Heart rate: Approximately 90 beats/min
2. Rhythm: Sinus arrhythmia
3. Axis: Not calculated, as only lead II is provided
4. P = 0.06 sec × 0.15 to 0.30 mv

   P-R = 0.1 sec

   QRS = 0.06 sec; remember, amplitude is not significant in the cow

   S-T segment and T wave = Most of the T waves are similar and 0.12 sec in duration. Notice that the T wave associated with the fifth and ninth P-QRS-T sequences (counting from the left) are smaller than the rest. Notice also that these two sequences also have slightly taller P waves than the others.

   Q-T = 0.28 sec
5. Miscellaneous criteria: Careful observation reveals that the fifth and ninth P-QRS-T sequences are associated with a longer R-R interval, suggesting increased vagal tone is responsible for a slight shift in the pacemaker. This was regularly repeatable throughout the entire ECG and was felt to be associated with respiration. The steady baseline would suggest that these minor variations are not due to artifact.
6. Technician action: There appears to be

no need for specific action with respect to this ECG. Most ventricular septal defects eventually result in signs of right heart failure in the calf. This particular calf had a concurrent respiratory infection, and a heart murmur was detected while listening to the lungs.

CASE 7-16 (Top Tracing)

1. Heart rate: The R-R interval is approximately 32 small boxes, which calculates to a rate of 94 beats/min
2. Rhythm: The R-R interval appears fairly regular
3. Axis: The axis cannot be calculated, as only lead II is present
4. P = P wave measurement is difficult because none of the P waves appear similar

   P-R = A precise P-R interval cannot be determined owing to variation in shape of the P + QRS complexes

   QRS = The first, second, and fourth QRS complexes appear to measure 0.07 sec × 2.1 mv

   S-T segment and T wave = No two are the same; therefore, they cannot be measured

   Q-T = No two are the same; therefore, they cannot be measured
5. Miscellaneous criteria: Close inspection reveals no two P-QRS-T sequences appear the same. In addition, bizarre "waves" appear immediately before the P wave of the first sequence, between the second and third R waves,

during the T wave of the second P-QRS-T sequence, immediately before the fourth P wave and just after the fourth T wave. In addition, the third QRS complex looks considerably different from the others, yet it appears to be preceded by a P and followed by a T. Note that none of these bizarre waves has any effect on the underlying rhythm. What is the problem? These bizarre waves are artifacts caused by patient movement, which distorts the shape of some complexes but cannot affect the rhythm. The lower tracing represents this patient's ECG free of artifacts.

CASE 7-16 (Lower Tracing)

1. Heart rate: Approximately 80 beats/min
2. Rhythm: Sinus arrhythmia; note the variation of the R-R intervals (P-P intervals) and the repetition of the sequence, which repeats itself with each respiratory cycle
3. Axis: Cannot be calculated
4. P = 0.05 sec × 0.25 mv

   P-R = 0.12 sec

   QRS = 0.07 sec × 1.9 mv

   S-T segment and T wave = Slight S-T segment depression is seen but this does not exceed 0.2 mv, which is the criteria for significance

   Q-T = 0.22 sec
5. Miscellaneous criteria: There are no "no" answers for the six important questions we ask when evaluating each ECG. Review these questions in Cases 7-1 through 7-10 if you need to.

6. Technician action: The proper ECG evaluation is that the top tracing is unreadable because of patient movement artifact. The lower tracing shows mild P mitrale (left atrial enlargement) with sinus arrhythmia. The proper action would have been to repeat the ECG, correcting for patient movement by adequate restraint.

CASE 7–17

1. Heart rate: At the beginning of the ECG, the heart rate is approximately 300 beats/min; at the end, approximately 150 beats/min

2. Rhythm: The first portion of the ECG is a very regular rapid rhythm (tachycardia), which abruptly slows to a sinus arrhythmia about two-thirds of the way across the strip.

3. Axis: Unable to calculate, as only one lead is present

4. P = Variable

    P-R = Variable, but last three sequences appear regular at 0.10 sec

    QRS = 0.05 sec × 1.1 mv

    S-T segment and T wave = Variable

    Q-T = Last four sequences appear the same, at 0.17 sec

5. Miscellaneous criteria: After examining this ECG by asking the six basic questions, "no" answers may be given to all six questions. Let's examine them in detail.

Question 1. Is the heart rate normal or abnormal? In the first portion the heart rate is very rapid (300 beats/min) and in the last portion it resumes a normal rate (150 beats/min).

Question 2. Is the rhythm regular or irregular? The first portion is regular; the second portion is irregular and different from the first portion.

Question 3. Can I identify P waves and QRS complexes? In the first portion it is hard to say where the P waves are, as only one wave is present between each R wave. Is this T, P, or T and P? At the end of the ECG, P waves can be plainly seen. QRS complexes are seen throughout the ECG.

Question 4. Is there a P wave in front of every QRS complex and a QRS complex following every P wave? In the last third of the ECG we can say "yes," but in the first two-thirds we must say "no" because P waves cannot be defined. What clue suggests they are there, however? Note the R waves appear similar throughout the entire ECG tracing. This would suggest that they are being formed normally, which would lead you to think that P waves must be hidden somewhere between each R-R interval.

Question 5. Are the P waves and QRS complexes consistently related to each other? Only the last three P-R intervals appear the same. Since we cannot define P waves in the first portion of the ECG, we cannot say whether they are the same or not. What about the P-R interval of the fourth P-QRS-T sequence from the end? Careful measurement shows this P-R interval is slightly shorter than the last three. Note that it is the first one following the rapid rate and it is preceded by a pause. This pause allows the A-V node a chance to rest for a brief moment, and the next beat is often conducted more rapidly than ordinary (super normal conduction). Note also that P wave is slightly smaller than the others. That too is common when a pause follows a rapid rhythm.

Question 6. Do all the P waves look alike and do all the QRS complexes look alike? As we have already said, the QRS complexes look similar throughout the tracing, but the P waves do not all look alike.

6. Technician action. When a very rapid rhythm is seen when the QRS complex appears to be fairly normal, a supraventricular tachycardia should be expected. Direct pressure to both eyes (ocular pressure) or massage on either side of the throat just proximal to the larynx (carotid sinus massage) should be performed. This will sometimes "break" or stop the pattern of tachycardia and allow the normal rhythm to take over. In this case, ocular pressure was applied at the beginning of this ECG, and it was successful in breaking the tachycardia. Fainting or syncope is common in patients with prolonged or sustained supraventricular tachycardia.

CASE 7 – 18

1. Heart rate: The rate of the normal-appearing P-QRS-T sequence is approximately 65 beats/min

2. Rhythm: The rhythm of the normal complexes appears to vary slightly (sinus arrhythmia) but the first two QRS complexes are followed closely by a bizarre-appearing complex, which is a VPC. Both of these VPCs have the same shape and are therefore considered uniform.

3. Axis: Cannot be determined

4. P = Slightly variable; 0.04 sec × 0.1 to 0.25 mv
   P-R = 0.10 sec
   QRS = 0.04 sec × 2.4 mv
   S-T segment and T wave = The S-T segment slurs into a negative T wave
   Q-T = 0.16 sec

5. Miscellaneous criteria: Note the small positive deflection following the first VPC. This is a P wave that was blocked from being conducted to the ventricles because the VPC depolarized the lower zones of the A-V node when it fired and not enough time has elapsed for those cells to repolarize and be ready to transmit the P-wave activity to the ventricles. This is called ventricular bigeminy with paroxysmal second-degree A-V block. The term "bigeminy" refers to the alternate sequence of normal QRS complexes and VPCs. A pulse wave is generated by the normal P-QRS-T sequence but usually none can be felt following

the VPC. If you were to listen to the heart with a stethoscope and simultaneously palpate the femoral pulse, you would hear two heartbeats for each pulse wave (2:1 pulse deficit).

6. Technician action: Remain calm. Remember, the first pulse to take in an emergency is your own. Ventricular bigeminy is commonly seen during the induction phase of IV barbiturate anesthesia. It is usually self limiting and disappears on its own within a few minutes. Note that the VPCs do not disturb the rhythm much at all. The patient's color, perfusion, respirations, and reflexes should be evaluated. The ECG monitor should remain attached to allow documentation of the return to a normal rhythm and surgery should be delayed until the normal rhythm has returned. If for some reason the bigeminy does not disappear or it progresses to ventricular tachycardia, IV lidocaine should be administered.

CASE 7 – 19

1. Heart rate: Only two R waves are seen. The R-R interval is 93 small boxes or 1.86 sec, which would calculate a heart rate of 32 beats/min; this is very slow for the cat.

2. Rhythm: With only two QRS complexes present, it is difficult to characterize the rhythm other than to note it is very slow (bradycardia); note that P waves are not visible.

3. Axis: Cannot be determined, as only lead II is given.

4. P = None visible
   P-R = Cannot calculate
   QRS = 0.05 sec × 0.7 mv
   S-T segment and T wave = The S-T segment is very long and lasts approximately 0.24 sec.
   Q-T = The Q-T interval is also prolonged, mostly because of the long S-T segment. It measures 0.40 sec in duration.

5. Miscellaneous criteria: It is most important to recognize that no P waves can be seen. When no P waves or undulation of the baseline (F waves) can be found at all, atrial standstill is said to be present. The findings in this ECG are bradycardia, prolonged S-T segment and Q-T intervals, and atrial standstill. Sixty-cycle electrical interference is also present, which may have affected our ability to see P waves. This is unlikely, however, as there is no variation in the 60-cycle pattern in the area where we would expect to see P waves.

6. Technician action: The combined presence of atrial standstill (no P waves), bradycardia (slow heart rate), and prolonged S-T segment and Q-T interval measurements should alert the technician to check for serum electrolyte imbalances immediately. Anesthesia should not be attempted until the electrolyte imbalance has been corrected and the ECG is more normal. This ECG is typical of hyperkalemia (elevated serum potassium) in the cat. The hyperkalemia is being caused by the urethral obstruction. The urinary bladder should

be emptied by cystocentesis (transabdominal needle puncture into the bladder and withdrawal of urine). IV administration of normal saline with dextrose at 1.0 g/kg and regular insulin at 0.5 μ/kg added to the saline solution should begin immediately. This will lower the serum potassium. Calcium chloride may also be used in place of the saline, glucose, insulin "cocktail" to lower serum potassium.

CASE 7-20

1. Heart rate: It is difficult to calculate the heart rate when there is such a variation throughout the tracing. The total time shown on this ECG is approximately 3.8 sec. If we rounded this off to 4 sec and then multiplied the number of complexes by 15, we could get a rough estimate of the heart rate (7 complexes $\times$ 15 = 105 beats/min).

2. Rhythm: The rhythm is extremely variable and irregular with a long pause in the middle of the ECG where no waves are seen. This is a period of sinus arrest (no P waves are formed) and it is ended by a QRS complex that looks rather like the remainder of the QRS complexes but without a P wave preceding it. This is a junctional escape beat and has been labeled "JE" to help identify it.

3. Axis: Cannot be calculated, as only lead II is present.

4. P = 0.04 sec $\times$ 0.15 mv; note that only two P waves can be clearly seen—one precedes the second QRS complex from the left and one precedes the next to last QRS complex on the right

P-R = 0.14 sec for the one on the left; 0.16 sec for the one on the right

QRS = 0.05 sec $\times$ 1.4 mv

S-T segment and T wave = There is considerable variation in the S-T segment and T wave although the first, third, fifth, and seventh look similar

Q-T = 0.20 sec

5. Miscellaneous criteria: The major problem in this ECG appears to be with the P wave as almost all the QRS complexes look alike. No P wave is seen before the first QRS complex. The T of the second sequence and the P of the third sequence are seen occurring together, forming a single M-shaped wave as the P of the third sequence occurs prematurely. Then there is a long pause where no P wave activity is seen (sinus arrest) that ends with the junctional escape beat. The next QRS complex appears to have a negative P wave as seen by the negative deflection immediately following the T wave of the junctional escape complex. The sixth P-QRS-T sequence appears almost normal except there is a small positive deflection in the middle of the S-T segment. This is the P wave of the last P-QRS-T sequence, and it occurs prematurely also. There is evidence to support that A-V nodal conduction is variable and is prolonged, as seen by the different P-R interval measurements. This ECG represents a condition seen in elderly schnauzers, dachshunds, and cocker spaniels called the sick sinus syndrome. Dysfunction of the sino-atrial (S-A) node, usually due to a deterioration in its blood supply, results in some periods of premature firing and some periods of no firing at all. This results in an irregular rhythm with long pauses in which no heartbeats are produced. It is usually during these long pauses that fainting occurs.

6. Technician action: These patients are usually somewhat weak and have an easily determined irregular heart rhythm on physical examination. Prompt recognition of the type of disorder causing this irregular rhythm is afforded by the ECG. Consequently an ECG should be recorded as soon as possible. When the sick sinus syndrome is suspected, an atropine response test is indicated. This is performed, following the clinician's approval, by injecting atropine IV at a dose of 0.01 to 0.02 mg/kg and recording the ECG over the next 5 min. In patients in which the S-A node is firing abnormally owing to excessive vagal nerve stimulation, the ECG will become rapid and regular (sinus tachycardia) usually between 1 and 2 min after the injection. In patients whose S-A node is firing abnormally because of disease of the S-A node itself, atropine will have little or no effect on the rhythm. In patients with elevated vagal tone and S-A node disease, atropine may increase the rate slightly, indicating a trial period of therapy with oral vagolytic drugs. In most cases of sick sinus syndrome, pacemaker implantation is the treatment of choice.

Index

Note: Page numbers in *italics* refer to illustrations; page numbers followed by t refer to tables.